# How to Melt Body Fat, Without Diets or Gyms

## The Busy Woman's Guide to Long Term Weight Loss, Rebooting Your Confidence, and Rekindling Your Youth.

**Adam Grayston**

# Table of Contents

# Introduction

At some point in every woman's life, issues and insecurities arise about their external appearance, and the usual go-to thought is, "I need to go on a diet or go to the gym." What if I told you that you will no longer have to waste your time on yo-yo diets or spending hours at the gym, but still manage to lose that undesired weight? You will not only avoid the extreme pressure of going to the gym every day (and feeling guilty about each day that you don't go) or the struggles of committing to a strict diet, but by using my proven method, you will still lose weight and keep it off for longer, or permanently for that matter. You get to choose when to fit exercise into your schedule, and the amount of times per week that you will follow this exercise routine. You don't need to become vegan, start juicing or even try the ever-popular keto diet; you just need to make healthier food choices and exercise part of your lifestyle. That sounds simple enough, doesn't it? The most exciting fact is that it is truly possible to lose weight in this way and cut through all the bullshit you've been told before about fat loss, so you can become the best version of you that's confident about their body shape. You don't need to make any drastic new year's resolutions or spend days or even hours preparing to start. Start where you are, no matter how insecure and demotivated you may feel at this very moment, because if you're waiting for the right time or the perfect moment, you'll be waiting for a very long time.

The sad fact of the matter is that 91% of women are unhappy with their bodies (Palmer, 2013). As a father to my four-year-old little girl Amber, this statistic scares me while at the same time motivates me even more to change the way weight loss and health is perceived. I know that there are millions of women out there who are still struggling to lose weight, and this motivates me to show them the easiest and most effective way to lose weight, for good, without dieting or visiting gyms ever again (I don't have anything against gyms, I love gyms, but they're not necessary to get great results). The dieting industry is doing more harm than good for women who want to shed weight. They all promise immediate results, no matter what the long-term negative effects might be. There are charlatans who may say that your weight will stay off even when you have stopped the diet, which is largely untrue. Most diets don't provide you with the entire truth, they just focus on losing weight fast and rarely in a healthy or sustainable way. They are not concerned with developing healthy routines or ensuring that your hormones are not damaged through rapid weight loss methods. Diets only work in the short-term. They're meant to help you lose the most weight over the shortest amount of time. They are a gimmick and trap women in a negative cycle as all the yo-yo dieting causes your hormones to store more body fat, think of it like survival mode, your body can store a little body fat each time it experiences heavy calorie restriction. This is the result of what you put your body through when dieting. Your body is put under extreme stress when your food intake fluctuates drastically, so it's natural defense to store some calories in case you start starving it again, so it creates extra body fat.

My mission is to show you the easiest and simplest way to lose weight and keep it off, without giving up your favorite foods or putting any unnecessary stress on your hormones. Life can sometimes get in the way of your health through: work, starting a family, relationship difficulties, bereavement, marriage, divorce, ill-health and the list could go on. I have been through all of these stressors in my life therefore, I know firsthand how life can get in the way of what you really want to do and, more importantly, what you really need. How you choose to handle what life throws at you will determine a lot of what you will achieve in the future. If you are reading this book, you have probably already tried out at least a dozen of these fad diets and they have failed, otherwise you would not be seeking an alternative.

I would like to dedicate this book to my daughter, Amber. I feel it's my duty help and re-educate as many people as possible with my work and this book, so that your generation, and many of the generations before you and after you, will live in a world where we see our health and wellbeing as an asset and not something to be taken for granted. I picture a world where most people are in good health in body and mind because they genuinely care enough about it and they're willing to make self-care more of a priority over their work or social commitments. Self-care doesn't need to take over your life, it just has to be part of it.

## Why Should You Believe That Any of This Is True?

I've been helping busy women lose weight for ten years now, since I first started my career back in 2011. I first qualified as a personal trainer, then I went on to study Science at the University of Central Lancashire because I wanted to understand exactly how the body works and the effects that the food we put into it our body has on our overall well-being and waistline. I've had the privilege of helping women from all over the world lose up to and over 20 lbs in twelve weeks through my online training program, *Women Who Conquer Transformation Coaching*. Some are busy mums and some are industry leaders in the corporate world, and I can help you too.

Helping women to lose weight (without dieting or gyms) is important to me because it will help you reboot your confidence, boost your daily energy levels, increase your productivity, maintain healthier relationships, and be genuinely happy. Weight gain can impact a woman's confidence and approach to life; they may put on a brave face and seem confident, but deep down, they are struggling because they just can't seem to shake off those extra pounds and break those bad habits. Part of my mission is to help women feel more comfortable in their own skin again, to smile when they see themselves in the mirror, and have no more body shaming. I want to help them make themselves, and their self-care, a priority again, instead of always putting everything and everyone else first. It's time for you to manifest the best version of yourself.

## Where My Passion Was Ignited

Throughout my childhood and teenage years, my brothers and I survived on microwave meals and pies most of the time as my mum worked long night shifts as a single parent. My mum was and still is a smoker (the generation that smoked in their houses and on airplanes, and I smoked for a few years as a teenager as most do at those ages along with my other friends). I wanted to be healthy, exercise, eat healthy food and be outdoors as much as I possibly could. As a child, I was also obsessed with martial arts and other sports. The moment after I finished high school, I was a full-time apprentice mechanic. This is when I could start to buy my own food; I opted for fresh meat, vegetables and fruit. I would also look up easy recipes to cook simple meals, and that's when my passion for healthy eating really emerged. Like most young adults, I was out on the weekends at the pubs and out partying. I still ate unhealthy food over the weekends because I knew I could afford to thanks to my exercise regime. I was eating well throughout the rest of the week, so why deprive myself of something that I really enjoyed?

When I had spare time between martial arts training, I would study nutrition. My life was centered around what I loved. I was living, eating, and exercising the way I wanted to, and this is when I found my true passion: eating healthy and getting regular exercise. I liked the gym, but I preferred training Jeet Kune Do and Brazilian Jiu Jitsu. I had no interest in improving my muscle tone or symmetry standing in front of the mirror, I exercised to become healthier, fitter and to improve my wellbeing.

When the recession hit in 2008, I was laid off from work. Over the next two and a half years, I went on to have eight different jobs in eight different industries. It wore me down mentally and physically. I was drinking heavily most weekends and not getting much exercise during the week. I wasn't eating well; it felt like my life was going nowhere. It was true, my life at that stage was not progressing in any way. So at the age of 23, I decided to enroll in college to become a fully qualified personal trainer. I loved everything about it. Once I was qualified, I wanted to soak up more information about the biology behind exercise and nutrition, so I signed up for a foundation science degree at the University of Central

Lancashire. This was the turning point in my life, as I was finally moving forward. I was happy again and once I had completed my degree; I went straight into the health and fitness industry—full-time! I dedicated myself to my new career working 6-7 days a week and picking myself up again after my life was at a dead end. I made the conscious choice to chase my dreams and turn my life around just like anyone else is able to do. You just need to want it enough, take the risk, make the leap, and do what you need to do to change your life for the better. I have a proven track record of clients who have been successful after following my program and I am positive that I can do the same for you.

In an article I had featured on Fox34.com, they asked me how I got to where I am today. The answer was simple: This year, I am celebrating ten years in the weight loss industry. I've been providing life-changing support to women who wish to reach their ultimate well-being goals. My mission is to help women melt away body fat and regain their confidence in the long-term, all without having to go to gym, go on hardcore diets, or use complex programs. I help women realize that while dieting may seem like the best solution for weight loss, these diets are actually doing just the opposite because they usually make you put on weight as soon as you stop following them. Diets are not the solution. In fact, diets are making people bigger, not slimmer! Many studies show that rather than losing weight, most women who diet often end up gaining weight in the long run. For decades, dieting has been the norm for women to shed unwanted body fat. This is completely understandable as many diet companies are marketing the tiny 5% exceptional and successful results of their clients yet, statistically, 95% of those women fail to keep the weight off in the end. Actually, these women end up putting on more weight, resulting in terribly low confidence, self-esteem, attempts to follow yet another harmful diet which induces "calorie restriction and loss of muscle mass that may cause your body's metabolism to slow down, making it easier to re-gain weight once you return to your usual eating pattern" (Spritzler, 2020, para. 31).

This is the main reason why I do what I do. I believe in the physical and mental benefits of healthy eating and various types of exercise. Instead of giving empty promises and potential long-term damage to your body (like with dieting), I provide long lasting results (both physically and mentally). I don't only want to see you lose weight, but I will help you create the habits you need to keep it off, keeping that motivation high and your confidence boosted. At any one time 50% of women are on a diet, and women that do diet programmes generally do around three a year. On top of that, one in three teenage girls have either tried to diet or considered going on a diet. So that just shows you how much diets, juicing, or detoxes, and weight loss in general is part and parcel of society, and a lot of it is aimed at women. A woman's body works slightly differently to a man's. They typically gain weight quicker and tend to carry extra weight because of hormonal reasons and having the ability to carry babies.

There are a lot of women who have grown up dieting. They have seen parents or other family members dieting, or seen other women dieting in magazines or TV, everywhere. There's billions and billions of dollars being spent promoting diets. There's a lot of information out there about weight loss and the vast majority of it you just don't need to know, thousands and thousands of web pages and articles on weight loss and food, but only a tiny percentage of that information is what you truly need to know. You sign up for weight loss programmes, weight loss groups, juicing programmes, detoxes, and get all these pieces of information but none of it is specific to you, and none of it tells you what you actually need to put in your body, how much you need, and how to make it sustainable.

Weight loss has become a billion dollar industry. "The U.S. weight loss market reached a record $78 billion in 2019, but suffered a 21% decline in value during 2020 due to the Covid-19 pandemic and recession" ("U.S. Weight Loss & Diet Control Market Report 2021," 2021, para. 1). The current misconceptions are: you cannot be simultaneously overweight and fit, all plus-sized women are unhealthy and should lose weight, everyone can lose weight if they just follow a diet plan, and the main reason that women regain weight is because they did not stick to the diet properly. Unfortunately, many don't do their research about all of the potential risks and pitfalls of dieting before you attempt to follow any of them. However, I have already done that research. I already have tried and tested my methods that work and sustain weight loss with my clients. I have put in the effort on your behalf, so that I can assist you to achieve your weight loss goals. I am invested in your success and will support you each step of the way, until you have reached your end goal and more than that, create a sustainable plan to extend beyond my program and for you to keep fit and healthy in the long run.

# Chapter 1

# No More Hopes and Prayers

*"There's this one color that I can see only when I'm daydreaming. It's probably just a pigment of my imagination."*

## Getting in Shape Is Not Rocket Science

The first step is to take deliberate action on what you need to do to get some momentum going. It is easy to daydream of a better life, a better car, house, or a leaner body; it is exciting and stimulating to fantasize about what we could achieve if we applied ourselves wholeheartedly. I have been guilty of this. I used to daydream all the time, I used to put things off if they're not urgent, or most times it was easier and more exciting to think about achieving a goal than taking action. The truth is, procrastination gets you nowhere, fast. We are distracted all the time, app notifications being the number one side tracker of our daily lives, checking likes, posting on social media, watching videos. Then we have our evening side tracker, Netflix, which is no longer "Netflix and chill" more like "get my Netflix thrill." Work emails are becoming a hot topic in recent press as more people want to avoid answering out of hours emails, another popular way of prioritizing work over our other needs or goals.

Procrastination is rarely about people being lazy, there are many valid reasons why people procrastinate. It could be the fear of failure, putting off tasks that you don't like, or feeling like you need to perform well at the task but you are not certain you will be able to reach the high standards set by you or others. Sometimes it doesn't need to be as complex as this, perhaps you are just simply exhausted after a hard day at work. It is easier to procrastinate when your goals are not specific enough or not clearly defined. We live in an age of instant gratification and want to be fitter, slimmer, and healthier *now*—not tomorrow, next week or next year. So, if our reward is delayed, we might procrastinate simply because we think we may never reach our end goal. You might have heard people saying, "That's my future self's problem." This is aptly connected to procrastination because if you think that having a healthier lifestyle is not imperative right now, you may not see the point in starting at all, until the future arrives and you may end up having to deal with health issues.

Many women put off taking action as they are waiting for something better to come along like the new fad diet, when they feel more confident, or when they have more time. What they don't realize is that this will all fall into place by just taking the first few steps. Or it could be a case of, "I'm only in my thirties, I will worry more about this when I'm in my fifties or sixties." Perhaps you are one of those people who always wait for something better to come along, or for things to happen at the "right" time, or there are simply too many options to choose from so they don't make a choice at all. You could feel anxious, overwhelmed, or the worst kind of perfectionist who doesn't start a task at all for fear that they won't do it perfectly. No matter what your reason is behind being a procrastinator, it is certainly possible to overcome these obstacles by being brave, making the decision, and taking the first steps forward you need to take in order to start your journey.

When taking deliberate action on your weight, starvation is not the answer. This method of dieting could potentially lead to eating disorders for some people, simply because your body was not made to function without any food (energy source). This is due to the similarities between disorder eating and dieting. "Disordered eating may include restrictive eating, compulsive eating, or irregular or inflexible eating patterns. Dieting is one of the most common forms of disordered eating" (National Eating Disorders Collaboration, n.d.). Dieting that requires you to restrict your intake of foods, then allow you to "binge eat" is particularly dangerous. Physiologically, your body adapts to the vicious cycle. Psychologically, you feel guilty about eating bad food so you starve yourself to feel better about yourself. If there is a sudden and huge drop in the calories you consume, your body goes into survival mode as mentioned previously, other common side effects of restrictive dieting are headaches, fatigue, loss of sex drive and feeling more out of breath than normal. Heavy calorie restriction can eventually lead to a breakdown of muscle fibres, which can be harmful and slow your metabolism down further. The best way to prevent this is to make small, sensible and sustainable changes to your eating habits to allow you to burn body fat without slowing your metabolism down or causing any of the other health issues.

The biggest obstacle to those who want to start changing their eating habits is the fear that they will never be able to eat any of their favourite foods again. When you cut something out of your diet, whether it's chocolate, a takeaway or alcohol it may be the only thing you can think about just because it is the very thing you cannot have. Thing about what happens when you take something away from a child that they really like, they get upset and they want it more, sometimes they'll even find ways to have it without you knowing if they can. Restriction or taking something away from a client has never been part of my method when I coach my clients, as they'll want it more and it's not a realistic approach that'll work in the long run. It's about making adjustments, and I'll show you what adjustments to make as we delve further into this book.

It is inevitable that life will be extremely busy at times, and it can feel like there are just not enough hours in the day. Thankfully, most people have at least a couple hours a day to do what they love or to use this free time more constructively. You can do an inventory of each day by breaking it down into what you have successfully achieved during that day, versus the time that you have wasted. Over the years I have encountered many clients, some who have been struggling to lose weight for over 10 years, or even for longer than that. There are various reasons for getting stuck at a certain weight or gaining that weight in the first place. You could have had a baby, gotten a new job, or had struggles that are so unbearable that it seems as though you have been to hell and back. There are far more reasons for weight gain and struggling to lose those extra pounds, but all of these struggles lead to the same results: You stop looking after yourself and put others' needs before your own.

During this time, we may become obsessed with the changes we want to make in our lives, but lack the motivation or confidence to take that first step towards change. We fantasize about being healthier, looking sexier, feeling confident in an outfit that we haven't been able to fit into for years, and having absolute confidence in ourselves. Hoping and praying for change is futile as we obviously need to actively do something about it in order to achieve the results. Our plan may be vague or meticulously mapped. We know what we need to be doing but we just don't do it. We see our weight loss problem as insurmountable or too difficult. We give up on taking action and resort back to just praying and hoping.

I am pretty sure that we have all made a New Year's resolution (many times). Commonly: "I'm going to lose weight, become fitter, and be healthier this year." The problem is that we all want to lose weight instantaneously, but that rarely happens so we just give up after a week or we do lose the weight but it returns as quickly as we lost it. There are far too many articles, social media posts, and magazines that promote "healthy" dieting. Many women have tried some of the hundreds of diets targeted to a certain aspect of your body. However, too many are left deflated and disappointed when they don't get the promised result, or if they've seen other people lose larger amounts of weight in the same time, they feel like they're failing because they're not getting the same results as others.

The truth is, it's not rocket science, it's a collection of small, effective changes and making sure that your expectations meet your reality. Your results and the speed of your results will be unique to you and there are several factors at play which you will come to understand by the time you've finished this book.

# Weight Loss Does Not Need to Be a Mountain

What if I said to you that weight loss will never be daunting again, it will be like climbing a flight of stairs? There is a starting point, an end goal, and you know exactly which steps to take to get there. It can't be that easy, can it? Yes, absolutely, as it has worked for a myriad of women time and time again. If the plan is personalized to your specific needs and what you want out of it, you find success at each step of the way. The key point is that you will have to prioritize it and take definitive action. Now I am not saying that you have to eat rabbit food, cut out alcohol, or that you can't treat yourself to a decadent dessert once in a while. Nor am I saying that you have to become a marathon runner or a CrossFit junkie who lives for training, and has no other priorities or interests in life. If that is your thing, I am not saying that there is anything wrong with being completely dedicated to exercise, but if this is the lifestyle that you lead, then this book is most definitely not for you.

With my method of weight loss, it is the small steps that matter, the small achievements and small actions that will make the difference. The ones you take action are the ones who will get amazing results. It doesn't matter how small these actions are, as they will all add up over time. You do not need to completely overhaul your life and routine to get leaner, healthier, and regain your confidence. If you have ever seen my video interviews with my clients, they always say how simple and easy it is to do when you take small steps each week.

To start out, have an honest look at your habits, your daily routine or the negative self and excuses you use. Take the smallest unhealthy habits in your life and change those first one by one. Exercise is often seen as a form of punishment for the extra slice of cake that you had, which is not the truth, exercise should become your go to therapy instead (it's not a miracle cure but it's a very powerful tool for self care and burning calories). The idea is to get some sort of exercise at first by doing something that you enjoy. It's important to get your body moving and reduce the amount of bad stuff you put into your body. Just because we are used to something and it seems to be comfortable, that doesn't mean it's necessarily good for us; it is just that we are stuck in our comfort zone. In essence, it comes down to taking an honest look at yourself and your lifestyle and figuring out the small changes that you can make. Be willing to do things in a different way. Look at your activities for the day and try to cut out the unhealthy ones. "I don't have time to exercise" is a common excuse. If you are working from home in front of a computer the whole time, make sure that you get up once in a while, and walk around the house, garden, or around the block to get some movement going in your body.

When it comes to changing your eating habits, if you are trying to cut down on a certain food then don't keep it in the house. This way, you won't be tempted to eat it as often and you'll have to go out of your way to buy it which is cool because you'll be eating good food most of the time. If you don't have a coach to hold you accountable, then have at least one person in your life who supports your weight loss journey to hold you accountable and keep you motivated, or a friend who will exercise with you, as this will help keep you on track initially. Having friends or family to hold you accountable is not good long term as it rarely works out, it's a weird dynamic that I still don't fully understand but what I do know, is that for long term results, you have to become consistent and self-sufficient at maintaining a healthier lifestyle without other people's input, over time. Make sure you set reasonable goals that are suited to you, and remember that things are not going to always go according to plan. Some days might not allow you to have the time to work-out or eat healthy meals, but having a few off days does not reflect on your progress.

There are many situations that could potentially hold you back from sticking to your plan. It could be your family, friends, yourself, a special holiday, work, or other emotional stress. For example, your partner could bring home a delicious, irresistible dessert, when they know, you are trying to watch your calorie intake. A friend could order a deep-fried meal when you are at a restaurant and go on and on about how good it is while you are sitting with a 'Chicken Caesar Salad' in front of you. You too can be your own worst enemy. You need to give yourself some leverage and be more flexible so that you don't feel like you are having to punish yourself. Your journey to becoming leaner, healthier and more confident is not going to be perfect and life is always full of challenges, remember that consistency will always win, not perfection.

When you are on holiday, the last thing you want to think about is tracking food and exercising, which is fair enough, you have to factor those times into your new habits. However, if you do neither of these things for long enough, you will break your healthy habit and end up having to start all over again.

When you are at work, perhaps you have packed a healthy lunch, only to find out that they are serving some delicious pastries and sandwiches at the upcoming meeting that day! You might feel too embarrassed to eat your salad while everyone else is indulging. There's no reason to deprive yourself or say no, as long as around 80% of the time you're eating well and if you're still working towards your weight loss goal you're inside your calorie goal for the day.

Here are some excerpts from some of my many success stories from the testimonial videos on my website, http:// www.*womenwhoconquer.co.uk/coaching*

Amy is a super busy working mom who has ditched the dirty diets for good. She lost 7 lbs, 6 inches from the waist and 4 inches from her hips within six weeks from my online coaching program. From dashing between offices and grabbing junk food on the go, she was able to shrink her waistline and boost her confidence by taking absolute control of her eating habits.

Clare had an impressive twelve week online transformation. She was a super busy, tired mum who had lost her confidence, and who had some dangerously low vitamin and mineral levels. Afterwards, she became an energetic, in shape, confident mum. With her now toned abs and a spring in her step, she has no intention of slowing down. Clare lost a total of 17lbs in 12 weeks

One of my clients, Luci, has the following success story:

> My body had been roughly the same for about a decade - pretty much since having children - and had grown to like it less and less with each new day. I avoided looking in mirrors and hated shopping for clothes, as my tummy and boobs made me feel more like an old matron than Marily Moroe. I hit 47 and realized that despite all my efforts (I cooked yummy home-made food, reduced my alcohol consumption and did regular exercise) nothing much changed. I glanced into the future and could foresee more decades of not liking how I looked. That's what made me pissed off enough to be prepared to invest in doing something different.
>
> If I'm honest, it was Adam's *before and after* photos that convinced me to give his twelve-week transformation program a go. His first call with me to figure out whether

I was ready to make some changes was very thought-provoking and different to other personal trainers I'd come across. I took a leap of faith and decided that if I wanted to feel differently about my body before Christmas (which was 14 weeks away) I'd have to do something different... and now! The weekly on-line coaching calls really kept me on track. Knowing that I'd have our on-line zoom call every week motivated me to keep going, completing his coaching exercises and committing to the training schedule which we agreed on together. He started off making very small changes, so small that I didn't believe that they would make a difference...but they did. Adam reviewed my training plan and progress and sent messages throughout each week, making changes where necessary.

As a vegetarian, I had believed my diet was pretty healthy but he discovered something that I'd never thought about which became the needle-shifter. I began to see noticeable progress - in my weight, shape and hunger levels. It's been a game changer. I've bought jeans a size smaller and new underwear. All of my clothes feel a little roomier. I've had to create new holes in my belt. I can barely believe it but my waist has reduced by 10 inches in 11 weeks...even though I still had my usual wine on a Saturday night. When Adam showed me my personal before and after photos - I was stunned into silence. I'm still stunned by my transformation. twelve weeks is definitely long enough to see and feel a transformation but some of the insights and behavior patterns that Adam has helped me imbed mean that I feel that I'm just beginning. Adam has helped me create a vision of my healthier, fitter, slimmer, sexier, more confident self, that I couldn't even imagine twelve weeks ago. Watch out world, here comes Marilyn Monroe.

Nathalie, another busy, working mum (who worked part-time and ran her own small business), lost 15 pounds in just over a month. She conquered her evening binge eating problem and lost more weight than she'd ever lost before! All with no dieting and no gym workouts.

It should be evident now that you need to stop hoping and praying, and actually just start taking some small action. Nobody else is going to do it for you. You are the one who has to take the first step, and have the commitment and desire to follow my guidance to get your results. As with all my clients, they have benefitted immensely from my guidance, but I can give them only that—guidance. You, like them, will need to be the one to put in the effort.

# Chapter 2

# Start Where You Are

*"Why did the can crusher quit his job? Because it was soda pressing."*

## Don't Be Discouraged if You Are Not Where You Want to Be

You have to start where you are right now, this is the very beginning of your journey. One of my favourite quotes is, "To achieve greatness, start where you are, use what you have, do what you can," (Ashe, 2015, para 1). I apply this to everything I do in my life because there is no point in waiting until the conditions are perfect—there is no such thing! More often than not, it is a way of avoiding the problems we have that we need to fix. We always put it off and say, "I will do it another day," or "I will get

started on it when certain things in my life are in place."
Why not start now? Be brutality honest with yourself
right now, what is standing in your way? You might be
stressed from work or unhappy in your relationship, or
maybe it is one of those days when everything seems to
be going wrong. Maybe your car has broken down and
it is going to cost you £1000 to fix, a £1000 that you
don't necessarily have. These are real life problems that
we all face, but none of these should hold you back from
putting just one small step of action towards a more
positive lifestyle.

The conditions for starting this life-changing journey
will never be perfect; they may even be volatile and every
little distraction may create the perfect excuse not to start.
However, all of my clients have started exactly where
they were when I started working with them. They were
unhappy with their bodies, they had low confidence,
they were stressed and hiding behind baggy clothes every
day to disguise their lumps and bumps. They were in no
way 100% ready to make changes, but they knew they
needed to start then and there, otherwise they never
would. There would always be an excuse about how they
wanted to wait until their lives got better, but that day
never came. It is comparable to buying a lottery ticket
when you have a one in a million chance of winning.
If you wait for everything to fall into place before you
take action, you will have a better chance at winning the
lottery than losing weight and eating healthier if you wait

till then. If your child or partner was sick, unhappy or in dire need of help, you would not just wish away their illness, you would do something to help them straight away. Why should this not be the same for own health? We are all far more helpful to ourselves and everyone around us when we focus on self-care at the top of our priority list, and not always sacrificing your own well-being for the sake of others (obviously not in this case where your child might be is sick). Self-care stops you from spreading yourself too thin, which lessens your ability to give your best to others and to yourself.

One great way to start where you are now is to ask yourself a few honest questions. How much spare time do I have to invest in myself? Am I willing to spend money on getting help to invest in my weight loss journey? So many of us have signed up to something that was free and never touched it, be it a month's free gym membership to a free sample of the latest perfume. Is there any valid reason why I can't start today? What is it that is holding me back from getting in shape, being happier and being more confident within myself, right now? Many people self-reflect, but it merely stays a thought; if you were truly serious about changing your lifestyle, you would have self-reflections questions and answers that you would write down. There seems to be more dedication to change when you actually see your thoughts on a page.

Write these questions down and write the answers next to them; answer each of them completely honestly, so you can confirm and allow your brain to register each of them. It will help you to evaluate precisely where you are at this moment in time in a straightforward way, and it will be in black and white so there will be less chance of being able to deny it or convince yourself that you are in a better headspace than you really are. Creating change in your life is never easy and if you are facing major obstacles, it is even more difficult, but you need to keep your end goal in mind and see past your current difficulties. See the small improvements each day as a step in the right direction and always celebrate your small successes.

I try to see obstacles objectively. When facing obstacles, you may be reluctant to accept your current state. Some might simply refuse to take any action at all, because they are focused on the end goal rather than simply taking the first step. Sometimes we are so stressed that we don't even think of trying to be more objective. There is good news though! It is possible to become more objective and not take things too personally, if we are conscious of it and if we are willing to change. We can rewire our brains by choosing to act or respond rationally and logically to our goals and writing them down. The more we do this, the easier it will become to see things objectively and make much wiser lifestyle choices. Lastly, many people compare their progress to someone else's, which diverts them from their own journey, you must stay in your lane, focus on your changes and results without comparison to others. Another thing that could hold you back is the way we think about the past. Viewing your past failures constantly can stop you from thinking in a positive way or having the confidence to change your life in the future. Everything in your past, whether good or bad, has shaped you into who you are today; it is useless to wish that your past had been different. This will take your focus off your plan as the present is all any of us have to work with. To elaborate on the fact that it is also useless to compare yourself to others, if you focus on your abilities and potential, and not on others, you will be able to use your time more effectively, and apply yourself more to the actions you have planned to take.

One thing that really put my health and my life goals into perspective, is those videos online of the elderly being asked what advice they would give to the younger generation, one of the most common themes is to ' take care of our health ' and ' be happy '. It's not just my knowledge and understanding of biology or body and mindset transformations that fuels my drive to take care of myself, I look to the older generation for a little guidance too, they've lived more than us and can provide us with some great advice that we can act on today too. I'm not saying that you should go around pestering the elderly when they're in the supermarket or doing interviews in retirement homes, but think about your future health and how you'd like to age.

Writing down honest answers to some brutal questions is a mind-altering technique. "Writing therapy is a low-cost, easily accessible, and versatile form of therapy," (Ackerman, 2021, para. 9). It has proven to be one of the best ways to confirm problems and solutions to yourself, for yourself and then to take the right action to make a change. It helps you to see things from a different perspective. Writing things down is a great way to make a fresh start with your life, including your weight, diet and confidence. Just as it might not be that easy to take that first step to make a change in your life, it might be quite difficult to take the first step when writing down an honest inventory of where you really are in your life right now. Here are a few things to keep in mind before you get started. It doesn't matter how fast or how much you write, you may take an hour to write just a few sentences or half an hour to write five pages, but as long as you are writing, that is what is important. When you are writing your list of questions and answers, make sure that you give it your full attention. Don't focus on how well you are writing, just let it flow, naturally. Write whatever comes up first and as if you are the only one who will ever read it.

> Rather than just write out your goals in a topline way, write at least a paragraph on how it feels to achieve your goal. Acting like you have already achieved your goal will start to connect the dots between where you are now and the steps you need to take to achieve your goals. (Acton, 2017, para. 4)

It helps to have a perfect understanding of your goals and why you have really set them. What will you gain from achieving them and what thinks will improve as you work towards and complete your goals (weight, confidence, energy levels etc.)?

I don't know about you but if I don't write down my goals, I intend to forget them or get more easily side-tracked. It helps you to make a true commitment and it also gives you a clear picture. You engage with them more in this way and are able to commit yourself to them more easily. You will get clarity on what you really want. It will help to inspire you (especially if you track your progress too) and you will have improved focus because your time management skills will develop.

## Nobody Gets Fast Tracked and Skips to the End

Once you know where you're starting from, everything else will gradually fall into place as you make small changes but, if you rush it, you will fail. Metaphorically, it is like wanting to cook a new recipe and just assuming that you have everything you need in the cupboards and fridge. With this knowledge, however, you still start cooking it, knowing that you are completely unprepared.

Keeping to the above analogy, you need the tools, the plan, the formula, and the knowhow to prepare for your weight loss journey. The tools in this case do not refer to any gym equipment as such, but the simple knowledge of how to start and what to start with. If you haven't been exercising at all for a few years, then the best idea is to start with walking or doing some sort of light exercise every week, then build on this when you have formed the habit and have successfully fitted it into your weekly schedule. There is no point in signing a gym contract, planning to go and exercise every day, twice a day, if all you've done is walk the dog every day for five years.

The tools you need are what you need in order to start the journey, not physical tools. This can mean accepting where you are in your life right now, having the motivation to take the first step, and simply having the willingness and a pinch of confidence to plan ahead. The plan is where I will come in, helping you to decide on what you want out of your weight loss journey, what you are comfortable starting with, and setting both short-term and long-term goals in order to be successful. I will help and motivate you to start where you are. Don't feel embarrassed that if the most exercise you have done in years is walking the dog. Life gets busy, we all know that, but I will help you make that first step and to decide on the easiest way possible to fit an exercise routine into your week.

You will hear what I like to call a "formula", several times throughout the book. It is repeated to reiterate that you need to constantly focus on calorie intake vs burning off calories (while still being able to enjoy your treats). This formula is like the recipe in my analogy. You will get the tools, the plan, the goals, and then you need to combine all of these elements to create a positive output. The recipe in this case refers to both the steps and goals for your exercise regime but also to your intake of calories in what you eat. Calories in vs calories out and regular exercise is a proven formula that has never changed.

So don't be like the person who starts to follow a recipe without even having all of the ingredients. Be prepared! Go to the store, buy exactly what you need and then, and only then, start to follow the recipe. So take your starting point, add a bit of exercise into your weekly schedule, make sure you don't take in more calories than you burn off and stick to the plan (we will look at exercise and calories shortly), don't give up and make sure you keep a steady pace in mind, even on the days that you don't feel motivated. Once you have formed the habit by following your plan each week, you are sure to feel good about the outcome. On the other hand, it's okay to miss goals. Most people don't do something one hundred percent perfect when they do it for the first time. You can't skip to the end of your transformation journey and miss out on the steps in between. While this is impossible, it would also reduce the amount of gratification that you will feel at the end, as hard work most certainly reaps rewards. Working hard towards your goals might not always be enjoyable at times or you could just be having a bad day, but it is imperative to get to where you want to be.

Another analogy that could be used is when we climb a flight of stairs. We can't get to the next landing unless we take the next step up. While we are on each step, it may seem monotonous, or even pointless at times because we feel as though we are getting nowhere slowly. It doesn't seem like the small steps are making any kind of difference at all, but how else are we going to get to the top? Remember, "big things could not happen without small steps we take" (Choi, 2020, para. 2). Growing up, I was always told that hard work would reap rewards, that it would set me apart from my peers, and make me more successful.

What defines a hard worker, you may ask? You can easily recognize a hard worker as they put a great deal of effort into their work, either physically, mentally, or emotionally. They put in extra-long hours, work at a high intensity and complete many tasks in a short period of time. They're diligent, consistent, and maintain high standards. They plan and organize their work to be as productive as possible. They take initiative, identify opportunities, and are independent. Most importantly, they thrive on completing what they start.

Working hard does not need to be unpleasant, especially in the context of this book, as you will have moments of focus and dedication but it is also alright if you are not in "the zone" all day, every day. Your goal is to focus on being consistent and having a growth mindset (creating habits, having a positive mindset and learning new skills to improve certain areas of your life).

# Chapter 3

# Be Realistic

*"A recent study has found that women who carry a little extra weight live longer than the men who mention it."*

## Set Attainable Goals

Have you ever encountered someone who constantly brags about how much exercise they do, and how well they eat? It makes you feel like a lazy couch potato who couldn't care less about leading a healthier lifestyle, right? I have felt like that many times, and my immediate reaction is to boost my ego by doing more exercise than them, eat better than they do. The fact is, that I am already doing enough and I couldn't give a rat's ass about anyone else's exercise routine or eating habits (obviously, apart from my daughter and my clients). I don't train as much as some people, I don't eat as well as some people do but I still get regular exercise each week and I'm consistently eating well, and that's all that matters to me and that's all I aim for with my clients too. The standard I set is realistic, effective and sustainable, so I've no reason to worry about what others are achieving or how healthy they are, and the same applies to you.

Do you really need to exercise five to six times a week to get in great shape and feel good about yourself? No! Do you really need to eat super fresh and clean to get lean? No! It's quite common for people when they have the inspiration to have a better lifestyle (usually in January) to go all out, put pedal to the metal, and with a rocket up their arse like they're heading for the stars. Then suddenly, they get burnt out and end up feeling like their efforts have failed or their body has failed them. Most of the women I have worked with have, at some point, had an all or nothing mentality when it comes to weight loss. They start their first week at 100 mph, they stop eating cake and chocolate, they pour their alcohol down the drain, they replace all the meat and junk food with fruit and vegetables (which will probably go bad in a few days anyway), and exercise as much as their bodies can take, all within the first week. The first few days are amazing but by the end of the week the fatigue sets in. Your whole body aches, and you start to feel overwhelmed by the prospect of following the same routine all over again next week. It becomes more difficult to get out of bed in the second week, and you're less motivated to follow your new-found healthy routine. You lack energy and start to crave some of the delicious food you just threw out. Not to mention the guilt over ordering take-out over the weekend, after vowing to never eat take outs again. Your motivation is starting to dwindle, quicker than a pint of lager turns to piss and the next thing you know, you are snacking on chocolates again, and having a glass of wine after work every night. Already, you have labelled yourself as a failure, all because you have pushed yourself too hard, too fast, and too soon.

## It's a Light Jog, Not a Marathon or Sprint

It is a nice thought to always be fully committed and have enough time to cook fresh, healthy meals, while still having loads of time to exercise and having the perfect amount of rest. You can imagine living your life almost like a pro-athlete or maybe even a lady of leisure. Sounds perfect, doesn't it? Yet, this ideal life can hardly ever become our reality. Our reality is sometimes completely the opposite of what we want for our lives. Keep in mind that in between all of your activities with friends and family and busy days at work, you still need to find time to get enough quality rest. The truth is that unless you are retired or semi-retired, it is impossible to live the life of a pro-athlete or a lady of leisure. The truth is that you will not be able to have a full-time life with major commitments and have the time to be a fitness fanatic, health freak and lean machine.

The reality is that life is busy and hectic at times. It's sometimes like spinning plates, being twice as busy, running on hot coals, being snowed under, or being up to your neck in it. It's like Groundhog Day (a common phrase used by people during this whole COVID problem). You know exactly what I mean by all this. Life can be a bitch at times; this is all nothing unfamiliar to all of us. It is not all doom and gloom, things can change if you really want them to, you just need to set very specific goals to work towards. So, with any goals you set, you must be realistic. I set two to three goals per week with my clients. These are super easy, straight forward goals. These goals are nothing complex or unrealistic, they are just small, effective changes. Goals shouldn't deprive you of the things you enjoy, whether that's your favourite food, family time, or nights out. They should be easy to implement, not take up too much time or effort and be sustainable.

If you are struggling to figure out what goals to set each week, don't worry! I've got some great guidance coming up in this book, so sit tight. One thing to mention, which links to the previous chapter, is that small goals should be easy to take action on so they're easier to accomplish and commit to each week. The less effort you feel you need to put in, the better you feel and the more driven you will be to continue on your journey to becoming a fitter, healthier, and more confident you! When it comes to setting long term goals ( could be 6 months or a year), you need to set goals that are important to you and add value to your life; this is how you will stay motivated to achieve them. They need to make sense in the bigger picture of your life, and they need to have high value when they come to fruition, otherwise it will be extremely difficult to achieve any goal, let alone life goals. Another reason why we only set 2-3 goals per week, is because if we set any more than that you will be thinly buttering your commitment and energy at once and potentially miss out on achieving those goals each week, which will once again leave you feeling like a failure.

*Mind Tools* also speaks about a SMART method of goal setting. Your goals need to be specific, measurable, attainable, relevant, and time bound ("Golden Rules of Goal Setting," n.d.). They speak of goals needing to be as detailed as possible, because if they are not, they will be easier to give up on. In the case of reinventing your life, you need to see the image of exactly what your new life will look like so that you can keep your eye on the end prize. To make your goals measurable, decide how many pounds you ultimately want to lose or how many inches or dress sizes you'd like to drop. When you keep this in mind at your next training session or when you are preparing your next meal, it can help you stay focused on your goal. Don't forget to celebrate the small victories and avoid setting your standards too high, your expectations must meet your current reality. This doesn't mean that you can't set slightly more challenging goals as you go along, just remember to start small. Do what you need to do so that you can get what you want. If you set goals that are relevant to the time and energy that you have available on a daily basis, then you are more likely to achieve them. Put a time frame on what you want to achieve on a weekly basis; you could even achieve them quicker than you expected.

As mentioned in the previous chapter, it is as important to write down your goals as it is to write down the answers to questions that may be stopping you from starting where you are right now. You can keep it as a reference to the reality that you are intending to manifest for yourself. Since this journey to weight loss, healthy eating, and increased confidence is long-term, it is sometimes too easy to get bogged down with continually thinking about the future instead of focusing on each small step that is going to get you there. Lastly, don't ever give up on your goals, or on yourself for that matter, the ones who fail are the ones who give up. Review your goals from time to time if you need to so that you can stay on track.

The purpose of setting goals on a weekly basis is to celebrate the small victories which will help keep you motivated. Maybe you know exactly what you want, how many pounds and inches you want to lose, but you may not know how on Earth you are going to achieve it. In the words of Pablo Picasso, "Our goals can only be reached through a vehicle of a plan, in which we must fervently believe, and upon which we must vigorously act. There is no other route to success." The first step is to map out your process on how you will get to where you want to be. Each step needs to be made with the outcome in mind and a specific purpose behind it, otherwise you are walking through life blindly. You want to be successful right? In this case there is the specific focus on reinventing yourself. The reason why some people perform better than others is because they have set clear goals and as they progress towards their end goal, they are flexible enough to adjust them as they go along, which will make it more likely for them to achieve their goals.

Each small success or victory that you achieve is a confidence booster and will help you to make the next step or to set the bar a bit higher next time. The more small steps of success you accomplish, the more confidence and motivation you will have to keep going. According to *Positive Psychology*, they believe that there are five principles of goal setting: commitment, clarity, challenge, complexity, and feedback (Houston, 2020). These are familiar tools that I also use when helping a client to set their goals. If you are not fully committed, it will be far easier to give up before you reach your end goal. You have to really want it and have a full understanding of how you are going to get there. It is like setting down proverbial arrows on the ground that you need to follow, and understanding the motivation behind each part of your path.

It is also all about timing. You can't set your goals and then have unreasonable timelines in which to achieve them—that defeats the whole purpose of setting very specific goals in the first place! You cannot just fast track your life to where you want to be. The last part, which is where I come in with my clients, is to get constructive feedback on your progress. When my clients see that we are progressing towards your goals, this makes them more confident to achieve them and to set more goals in the process. This forms a vital part of the reflection process which I do with my clients each step of the way. You can do this yourself maybe once a week and just spend 10 minutes in a quiet place thinking about what you've achieved and what you will focus on for the following week, or even better, write it down.

# Chapter 4

# Priorities

*What's a horse's top priority when voting? A stable economy*

## Life Gets In the Way

Life is ever changing and evolving. Maybe you've changed careers, had a few setbacks, decided to start a family, and somewhere along the way you have lost part of yourself. This is because you stop making your own needs a top priority (or at least move it down towards the bottom of the list).

Quite often when I work with a client, they'll say on our call, "I don't feel like me anymore. I want the old me back." They've usually sacrificed a lot of time and energy into other areas of their lives like family, work, and other commitments, so they stop taking proper care of themselves and don't give their emotions or their bodies the attention they deserve. Life can pass by in a heartbeat (it's fleeting). Before you know it, it's Christmas again and another year has passed where you've ignored your own needs once again. You are still stuck in a negative cycle, wishing you were healthier, and wishing you'd made a few small changes. When looking back at the 365 days that have passed, you realize that you did have the time, you did have the energy, but you left yourself at the bottom of the list again.

It's easy to overlook your own needs, but it comes at a high price. If you're not taking good care of yourself, you can gain weight, lose your self-confidence, energy levels drop and your self-esteem is almost always negatively affected. Relationships can start to deteriorate and productivity at work can slow down. You might not even realize it at first. It can trigger a whole host of health issues. You can feel like a different person that you don't want to be and lose your zest for life.

## Self-Care Affects Every Aspect of Your Life

Self-care isn't something that you can buy or ask someone else to do for you. It starts within, within ourselves. You can be guided and coached but ultimately, you have to put in the work yourself. You have to make your own health and wellbeing a priority. In order for you to start caring about yourself, you need to find the time and put in some effort. I've had many occasions in the past when partners or relatives have contacted me concerned about a partner or family member, asking me if I'd be willing to help them because they haven't been looking after themselves properly and they don't know what else to do. This shows that it's not just the individual that's feeling the impact of neglected self-care, it's people close to us too. Unfortunately, I can't help them at that stage when it's the partners or relatives getting in touch, the person who's struggling HAS TO TAKE THE FIRST STEP to accepting they need help by actively looking for help, by contacting me. When that happens, you know that that person is sick and tired of their situation so much that they're ready to seek a solution, not a quick fix.

During my twenties, I spent around two to three years thinking that I was living life but I was actually going nowhere. At the time, I was in between jobs, working all day when I did have a job, watching TV at night and most days if I wasn't at work and drinking on the weekends, I lost the desire to stay in shape and focus on my own needs. I wasn't fit or healthy, I was just getting by. I used the 2008 recession as an excuse not to move forward or concentrate on any self-care. It wasn't until I got fired from a job for not turning up one day that I realised I was my own worst enemy and that I was standing in the way of my own progress. Sometimes you have to be at your lowest to take action and start looking after yourself. Chances are that you're at a low point and there's things you want to change and it's one of the reasons you bought this book. What you need to do now is be fully committed to your goals and take action. You need to start focusing on your self-care *today*, not Monday, not after your holiday, not when your kids grow up. You need to start today and end the bullshit story you keep telling yourself as to why you can't move forward and take some control of your health and wellness.

The attention that you put on your well-being, both physically and mentally, will affect every area of your life. For example, if you're exercising regularly, you'll be in a good mood and feel energetic. It affects your interactions with people, how you respond to situations and your general approach to life. When you feel at your best, you can have the best days. On the flip side, if you've ever been low on energy, sluggish and have decreased confidence, then the chances are that the opposite can happen. You may find it hard to get through each day, you regularly feel drained and begin to get a little short or snappy with people around you. It could be that you're not as extroverted as you used to be because your confidence is low and you don't have the energy to be as outgoing as you might have been.

How you feel and how well you look after yourself will have either a positive or negative impact on everything you do. No matter if you're out shopping, at home, or at work, your physical health and mental well-being is part of the equation. It can be the difference between having a good day or a bad day. Naturally, there are many things in life that can potentially throw your health and well-being off course, and they will succeed sometimes, but you need to build a robust, healthy body and mind to make sure that you can feel at your best most of the time.

It will of course, take clear action and time from you to consistently make yourself a priority. It won't happen overnight as most things never do, but you would be foolish to leave things to fate, or hope and pray that you will feel better without taking any action. So how do you go about making yourself a priority so that you can take the action needed to improve your life? Have you ever made a whole list of New Year's resolutions and not fulfilled any of them, or you lose interest in them a week in? You start to feel like a failure as your good intentions to build a more positive lifestyle have faded as fast as you have started acting. According to *Zoella*, there are twelve suggestions that I read which are very practical and effective techniques that anyone can start doing today . You can make time for you, speak kindly of yourself, get rid of the guilt, stop saying "yes" to everyone, love the skin you're in, don't be afraid to ask for help, let go of things you cannot control, tell yourself that you can do it, embrace your emotions, surround yourself with positive people, start a gratitude journal, and know that you're enough.

At some point during each day, you need to make time for yourself. Just take a break for a moment and rest. Do something that you love, like walking, reading, or whatever it is that you are interested in, even if you can only spend fifteen minutes on it. It needs to be something that will slow you down and briefly take you away the fast-paced rat race world we are living in. Try not to beat yourself up about things that you might not get done during the day; you don't need to tick off absolutely everything on your list every day. Just as you prioritize your tasks at work, you need to prioritize your self-care because your boss or your partner isn't going to do it for you, it always starts from within. Don't feel guilty about taking time to focus on your own needs. It's important to look after yourself for a change and not always place others' needs before your own. In many cases, the clients I work have developed a habit over time of becoming people pleasers and say "yes" to every request for help, every invite to social events or extra hours at work. Sometimes you need to do what you want to do. This might make you feel selfish or guilty at first, but you will be much happier for it in the end as you're applying a little TLC to yourself on a regular basis without feeling the need to please anyone.

In this book, we are focusing on how to improve your appearance and health, but it's just as important to learn to love yourself, despite what you may deem imperfect. "You can't control the past, the future or how other people perceive you and the sooner you make peace with that, the happier you'll be" (Zoella, 2020, para. 10). Be positive and even be your own cheerleader if you must, so that you can get to where you want to be, not forgetting that you will have both positive and negative emotions along the way. Learn to take the good with the bad. This includes making decisions about who you spend your time with. If you have friends or acquaintances who constantly talk about everything in a negative way, then reducing your time around and spending more time around positive people will improve your wellbeing and your focus. I know that last statement will ruffle some feathers, but it's true, the people who you surround yourself with will have an impact on your life, as tomorrow is not a guarantee for any of us, we must spend that time with the right people as best as we can.

Life is difficult enough as it is. If you are trying to keep positive about your plans to improve your life then surround yourself with like-minded people who understand and support your goals. When you take that time out each day, start to think of all the positive things that might have happened in your day (no matter how small they may seem) to boost your happiness. Writing them down and journaling will be helpful when you are having a bad day and are clouded with negativity; it may help you to see the positive parts of your current day by looking at what you have been positive about in the past. Lastly, you need to remember that even if your plan is for self-improvement, meet yourself each day with an empathy and warm towards becoming the new and improved (and ever improving) version of you. Many of the thoughts, steps, or actions that you take, will either move you away or towards your goals.

Self-care is about is caring for your own well-being which in turn will mean you can be more effective and helpful to those around you, especially your loved ones. As I've written this book which is during the Covid-19 pandemic, there has been a dramatic global increase in anxiety and depression. It is understandable as one of our basic needs is to interact with others socially and be able to spend time with others face to face. However, due to the many lockdowns implemented over the past year, this has limited social contact for every one of us. Due to being in the same environment and not being able to make a clear separation between work and home life (many of us having to work from home), some have begun to experience cabin fever. Isolation from others is anything but normal, yet we have all had to endure this in some shape or form since the dawn of the pandemic. It is understandable then that many more cases of anxiety and depression have emerged. It is vitally important to take care of your physical and emotional well-being as best you can. The starting point to self-care is being more aware of your physical and emotional or mental well-being.

Self-care is not only about focusing on your everyday habits and improving on these things. Your focus is on creating a healthier lifestyle and being able to appropriately deal with stress. The more effectively we can handle stress in our lives, the better we will cope under pressure; this will filter into every aspect of our lives, making it easier to focus on self-care and be better people, holistically. If we take a moment to focus on our health, it is not only about eating healthy and exercising regularly, but also about our general health care needs like going for regular basic screenings (like mammograms), having due diligence for getting the necessary vaccines, or, on a more basic level, actually going to the doctor when we feel sick instead of wishing our illness away and then end up taking those prescribed drugs anyway. Listen to your body and take the steps needed to nourish your body by using these methods.

According to *Everyday Health*, there are three basic categories of self-care: physical, emotional, and spiritual (Lawler, 2021). Physical care, which is a great starting point, involves eating nutritious food, getting weekly exercise in, and getting enough sleep. If you make this your starting point, it is sure to boost your emotional and spiritual well-being. Emotional care could range from meeting up with friends, taking a long walk alone, or not doing things that are going to cause unnecessary stress checking your emails after you've finished work or cracking open the booze knowing it's going slow you down the day after and stick to your hips! When it comes to your spiritual well-being, you don't have to become a religious zealot. It will be helpful to be kind to others, write down what you are grateful for, or just immerse yourself in nature for a while. It doesn't cost a thing to look after yourself in this way; it is all about finding something that you enjoy which allows you to calm your body and mind and doing that very thing as often as possible, which results in feeling fulfilled. Simply going out into the warm sunshine could have a similar effect and won't cost you anything. Self-care is what will bring you joy and is related entirely to your own needs. These actions should not just be temporary, because the aim of this book is to foster self-improvement and to help you create a happier, healthier life, long term.

According to widespread research, it is believed that the following self-care practices will lead to a longer life: taking up regular exercise (even light exercise will be beneficial), finding your true purpose in life, incorporating healthier meals into your weekly plan, getting sufficient sleep and spending time outside surrounded by nature. There's very strong evidence that links a lack of sleep to weight gain in both young people and adults. Many times on social media I see motivational videos or posts around how someone might work 7 days a week or they haven't taken any time off in 5 years all in the pursuit of success (just as an example). Yet many of the same people, from what I've seen online also talk about burnout and poor health from their exhaustive habits as though it's something to celebrate or admire. Lack of sleep and pushing our bodies to extremes overloads our bodies with stress (poor sleep being a factor of stress) and our immune system can start to deteriorate over time, so we become sick or unwell more often. Lack of energy, poor sleep, low libido, poor concentration, weight gain and in some cases anxiety and depression, all from poor self-care and treating our bodies like a tool rather than a living thing that should be nurtured not neglected. I can bet you probably know someone who fits into those the last few sentences, or maybe you know all too well for yourself what it's like too?

If we now bring our focus onto your mental well-being, according to *Mind*, they suggest the following six tips to follow when exercising self-care for your mental health. They advise that you should stay aware of your mental health, nourish your social life, try peer support, make time for therapeutic activities, look after your physical health, and if you feel that you may have a chronic mental condition, contact a healthcare professional as soon as possible. If you remain aware of your mental health, one of the imperative focuses you should have is on building up your self-esteem. Try some of these methods; start with the ones that resonate with you, such as: being kind to yourself, looking after yourself, looking out for the good things in your life, building a support network, going for talk or art therapy, learning to be assertive, setting yourself concrete challenges, and finding the necessary support for your specific needs. It might be useful to first think about what you value in life and what makes you truly happy.

Develop positive self-talk and don't compare your life's journey to anyone else's. Be sure to notice the small victories or successes that you have and give yourself credit for these. Accept compliments given to you, especially when you have achieved something either great or small. It might even help to write down a list of the things you like about yourself and build on these positive attributes. Remember that you can't combat all your life's problems at once, so focus on one thing at a time. Also, if something no longer serves you, give it up. Say "no" to things that you don't feel you can take on at the moment or to those negative people who you know will be a buzzkill to the improvements you are trying to make.

Self-care starts and ends with you, you don't need to approach this at full speed and full capacity at each moment of every day, remember that its not a sprint, or a marathon, it's more of a light jog and if you pace yourself properly, you're much less likely to fall off track because you've overdone it.

# Chapter 5

# The EASE Method

*"Why did the banana go to the doctor? Because it wasn't peeling well."*

## Make Body and Mindset Transformations Attainable

Does this conversation sound familiar? "I've tried every diet under the sun. I've done the shakes, done the detoxes, tried going to gym with my friend, but when one of us starts to quit, we both quit! I don't know what to do. There is so much information out there about food and weight loss that I don't know which to follow or what to believe. What is the right thing to do?"

Most of the conversations that I have had with potential clients over the past ten years have followed a similar dialogue in some shape or form. I realized very early in my career that information overload about weight loss was a massive problem for people. There is so much information out there, like in magazines where celebrities are pushing 30-day fixes. Every diet company has got a social media presence too, so you are always bombarded with mostly useless information about weight loss. I knew that the process to actually lose weight and keep it off was straight forward, it just takes the elements of guidance, support and accountability to connect it all together and make it work long term. It's inevitable that some of you reading this are very self-motivated individuals who can connect the dots to most things in life and make them work for you, whereas others need the three elements I just mentioned to help build a foundation to which you can flourish with your health and weight loss goals, self-sufficiently.

Diets are like alcohol. There are people who regularly use alcohol to temporarily take away some stress or pain . Just like a diet, this type of drinking gives the person temporary relief, but it doesn't get to the root cause of the pain or stress. I realized that many people who dieted just wanted the easy way out, the shortcut to shed a few pounds and feel better about themselves. They hoped that this would somehow trigger a commitment to keeping the pounds off, but, as most people know, diets are a recipe for failure as only a very small percentage succeed in starting a diet, sticking to it, and keeping it off by spontaneously developing healthy habits. That is the reason why there is a huge emphasis on having accountability and support, so that when my clients have a bad day or bad week, they get that accountability and support that they need to get back on track.

"Changing how you think is hard. Changing your environment isn't. By training your environment, your habits follow" (Andrews, 2021, para. 1). That sounds simple enough, doesn't it? It is more difficult to change your thought pattern than your environment as most of the time our thoughts are like automations, subconsciously following a habit that we have formed. For example, if you've ever taken a new job somewhere, it's all alien to you if you've never been there before, it takes quite some time to settle in to get to know your surrounds and the people you work with. If however, you're adjusting or improving on the job you have, it feels easier and more fluid to incorporate new things or new ways of doing things because you're already familiar with it. In this simple example, it is easy to see that when you change your environment, you have to put a lot of thought into even the most menial tasks. This can be applied to the way in which you approach your body transformation. So to keep on your journey of transformation, it is important to set up an environment conducive to your intended lifestyle change and not try to turn your life upside down suddenly. We're talking about small adjustments that can become familiar to you very quickly

Some other useful tips, according to *Precision Nutrition*, are: use smaller plates, don't keep food you are trying to avoid close at hand, park your car as far away as possible from the mall or store entrance so that you can walk a bit farther, have your bike ready so you can use it as your mode of transport, or get a breed of dog that you will have to walk often, so you can keep your body moving (Andrews, 2021).

One of the important parts of these changes is to acknowledge the progress you are making and remember that there will be many moments where you will feel uncomfortable. This is because you are going against what your body and mind is used to. As you progress in your transformation journey, we always aim to start slow and finish fast. Trying to change your physical appearance by changing your habits might seem difficult but being unhappy and not doing anything about it is more difficult to deal with. Many days, you are not going to want to work out at all, some days you are going to hate it before, during, and after, but that's the worst case scenario. There will be many days that you will feel motivated and elated afterwards. Although your effort needs to be consistent, the results might not be. Human beings are unpredictable. We are not machines, so we cannot expect our ever changing physiology to cooperate with us when we give our system a shock by finally exercising after decades of laziness. There will be sacrifices to be made and fears to be faced, but you will look back and realize that it all paid off, that you are better for it.

The only workout people regret is the one they never do!

What may help tremendously is to look at your situation like giving advice to a friend whom we love dearly. This will not only help you love yourself more but will also help you be kinder to yourself. Sometimes the advice you give to others is better than the way you've convinced yourself you have to go about it. There's the age old idea that it's sometimes far more difficult to follow your own advice, which may be excellent advice at that. We all need to stop limiting our minds and be open to change and learning something new that could transform our lives. You can do this by trying to put aside your prior knowledge of how to change your behavior and your old, preconceived ideas about it. It is all about perspective. Think about how you see yourself in relation to your environment and envision how things could be different (in a positive way). When you wake up each day, be more conscious of each action that you take throughout the day and how your decisions impact your wellbeing; this will make the process far easier. Do not get stuck in the rut of thinking that it is impossible for you to change, our lives are organic, and they should be ever changing, always evolving, and never stagnant.

You will be more successful if you truly believe that you are able to change the way you think, the way you eat, the way you exercise, and the way you approach self-care. The way we think has a direct effect on how we act, which can lead to either the right or the wrong outcome.

Thus, if you push yourself out of your comfort zone and consciously think positively about your life, it will certainly lead to the right outcomes. The goals you have set will come to fruition and the best version of yourself will emerge. If you believe that you are not a sporty person and now you have to force yourself to exercise, the likelihood that you will fail at sticking to an exercise program will be elevated, and it is difficult to get back onto that metaphorical horse and start again after going through failure. Believe you can make small adjustments, believe that feeling good about yourself is a god given right, believe that the person you are now is not going to be the same person tomorrow, or at any stage in the future. You don't have to be sporty or into the gym to get into great shape and to think otherwise will only hold you back further.

If, at any point in your twelve-week transformation process, you begin to compare yourself to others, stop for a moment and remind yourself that everyone's journeys are different and that there are a multitude of factors that allow each individual to progress and end up closer to their end goal. Your body shape, physical makeup, initial mindset, starting point (you could have started at a level of fitness far lower than another person in the first place), and the way in which you approach your goal will be different from the person to which you compare yourself to. It will be far better to have a growth mindset, where you believe that you are able to change, progress, and reach your goals through progressive mindset growth. These people truly want to evolve and improve themselves; they are willing to accept constructive feedback, making it possible for them to be open to leaving their comfort zone and trying something new. This kind of person is more likely to make the changes to their lifestyle and develop new habits despite any setbacks that they may face and overcome.

You need to set aside past failure and press forward to enable the change to take place. It can be overwhelming at first when it feels as though you are facing a mountain in front of you and think, "Is this actually going to work? Is it truly possible for me to get into the habit of healthy eating and weekly exercise?" It might be overwhelming at first but the most important step that you can take is the first, small one. The rest should then follow naturally. As you see the changes start to happen, you'll gain more confidence in taking the next steps. Past failures will dissipate as you move forwards. At this point, you could also use the lessons you have learnt from past failures as a catalyst to keep on changing and emerging into the person you aim to become.

My method of losing weight is simple, and the actual science behind losing weight is also just as simple, but diet companies hone in on these simplistic ideas and try to reinvent the wheel with very unnatural methods, then they pump millions into advertising and marketing their diets just because they have a lot of money to do that.

This has clearly had influence and created unhealthy, damaging trends for many generations. These companies have also overloaded everyone with information about the wrong ways to eat and lose weight. As soon as the internet was introduced and social media took over, we now have 10,000 times more information than we actually need, and definitely didn't ask for.

I've used the exact same method, helping women all over the world to lose weight for ten years now, but I didn't have a name for it, I just did it. I never really explained the process to my clients, they just came to me and we got straight to work. I realized that my method was even more effective with my online clients as they didn't have to take the time to see me face to face each week in order to complete their exercise, but they still got the guidance and support from me on a weekly basis. I give them advice on lifestyle changes, nutrition, exercise, and maintaining a positive mindset. It was a lightbulb moment for both me and my clients that this program was so effective online.

## Losing Weight and Building Habits to Keep the Weight Off

I decided that I had to give my method a name, so that I could explain how simple it is and also for my own peace of mind, so I named my method, The EASE Method. With my EASE Method, we first start with Evaluation and aims. As Steve Jobs used to say, "If today were the last day of my life, would I want to do what I am about to do today? If the answer is 'no' for too many days in a row, I know I need to change something." This is where I evaluate exactly where my client is right now in terms of lifestyle, health, mindset, and goals to change these aspects in their lives. For example, they might want to lose 20 lbs, drop a dress size or two, feel more confident about themselves and their bodies, and have more energy to be more productive at work or keep up with their kids.

The next step in my method is Accountability and support. Everyone has a plan, until life punches them in the face. It is essential in this step to provide each client with a means to have accountability and support so that they can stick to their plan each week. Even if life has thrown them lemons, we figure out the problems, make some lemonade and continue to work towards their goals. Why is accountability so important? Because one thing it does is it teaches you to take responsibility for your actions towards your health. Many people thrive on accountability, in university you have your lecturer or professor, in martial arts you have a coach or teacher, you have someone to answer to as you move forward towards your goals. It also helps you to take ownership of your actions so that you don't blame those around you or other things in life when things don't go according to plan. Holding people accountable is also a way of supporting them, they know they have someone to guide and support them throughout the journey no matter if they've had a good week or a bad week, and without judgement. Measuring your progress is simple when you are held accountable, which leads to the next part of my method of transformation.

The S in my EASE Method is for the plan and exercises being Simple to understand. To be a great expert, you have to be able to explain something in simple terms to those who are not experts on the subject, especially with all the confusing information out there on weight loss. It is important to know what you need to do to get great results. I explain this in simple terms, not by using all the science jargon that you may not understand (as much as I love to understand the body on a deeper level, it's not necessary for you to know all of it too in order for you to get amazing results). Lastly, the plan, method, or programme should be Easy to implement. It should feel easy to make changes to your weekly routine and habits in order to start losing weight. The easier it is to make small adjustments, the better you'll feel and the more driven you will be to achieve your weight loss goals. In this way, you will develop better habits to keep the results long term. I only set two to three small goals a week with each client, nothing more but sometimes less.

That is literally my methodology in a nutshell; these are the four pillars that make up my coaching program that I use with each client. I don't know why it took me all these years to write this down but I have my coach, Tim Drummond, to thank for this as he is the one who helped me become the coach I am today. That's right, I've been coached (several years of coaching in total, most of that with Tim) I've been in a position similar to my clients, having goals I wanted to achieve and needed some expertise, a plan and some accountability. Coaches have coaches too, there's no such thing as a one person success, there's almost always more people involved.

Chapter 6

# What Results Do You Want?

*"Why can athletes lift more than prisoners? Because the pros outweigh the cons!"*

## Be Clear About What You Want

Ask yourself this question: What results do I want? Do you want to lose 10 pounds, 20 pounds, 2 inches, or maybe even 10 inches? Do you want to feel more energetic each day and feel confident when you look at yourself in the mirror?

To have a clear vision about what you want, you should always keep the end result in mind each step of the way. This will help you to stay motivated with your goals and enable you to push through, no matter what adversities may come your way. Write your goals down and even put up little notes around your house in places that you will see often, if this will help you to remain focused. Some people find that putting together a vision board of goals or an old picture of you in shape or even out of shape as a reminder of your mission is something that really helps with motivation. This is why it is important to have a clear vision of what you want and where you want to be. This might be difficult to believe but there is actually a big difference between a vision and a goal. Your goals give you direction but your vision is where you want to end up, which is absolutely the case when it comes to following my program. My method is to help you set those goals (give you direction) after you have decided where you want to be (your vision). You need to set smaller goals that lead you to your big goals. This means setting up small daily, weekly, and monthly goals that will keep you on the path towards your vision. It seems pretty obvious to say that if we do what we should do, we will get the results that we are aiming for. However, the fact of the matter is that if you are not willing to put in the work, there is absolutely no way that you are going to achieve any goals or see any change, especially not the change that you have envisioned for yourself.

An alternative approach is to start to appreciate having a system in place and acknowledging the benefits. This is because "when you fall in love with the process rather than the product, you don't have to wait to give yourself permission to be happy" (Clear, 2018, para. 13).

It's always process THEN outcome, it's never the other way round otherwise our lives would be a complete mess. When you enjoy the process, it means you will attach good feelings/emotions to what you're doing which naturally encourages you to stick with it, long term. After you have put in all the hard work to achieve your goal, what then? What is left for you to focus on? This is an interesting perspective as this may lead you to going back to your previous lifestyle as you have now ticked that goal off your list. Remember, my program focuses on achieving goals, and, more importantly, to sustain your new habits to keep that weight off. During the 12 weeks, you should work on refining your goals and plans to improve your processes and chances of achieving them each week. This means that the process, rather than the goal, may be the more important factor here. There is always the misconception that once you reach a certain point in your life or once you obtain the certain material object that you have been saving up for, then you will be happy. Setting goals may give you an unrealistic sense that you will not be happy during the process of reaching your goal but only once you get to the finish line. You might see happiness as something that you can only enjoy in the future but that entails that you are missing out on many current happy moments in the process. For example, goals could be seen as something that you either achieve or you don't, and even if you do achieve them, it results in short-term happiness. My program takes you a step further as it is based on how to lose weight and keep it off, thus leading to long term satisfaction. When you know that weight loss and improving your health will have a positive effect on many areas of your life, you will want it to be part of your life, long term as an asset.

I have rarely worked with a client whose only goal is weight loss, there is almost always more to it. You may be sitting there thinking, "I don't know, I just want to lose weight." If you think for a little while longer, think about the positive impact weight loss will have on you. Will losing the weight you want to make you feel more confident with and without your clothes on? Do you want to start making yourself a priority again, instead of putting everyone and everything else first? Maybe as you have become older, you've realized that your energy levels are dipping and your clothes are getting tighter. You don't want to become the party pooper and be the first to go home to fall asleep after a few hours. And having to buy the next dress size up will no doubt bring up some negative emotions. A key question from me, is "what has led to the weight gain? ", for some it can be relationship difficulties, bereavement, change of occupation, low sense of worth, starting a family or sometimes the home environment which people grow up in (we tend to overlook the environment we grow up in as a factor in our future health and decision-making, yet it can affect many areas of your life as we grow older).

## Are You Fully Committed to Achieving Your Goals Right Now?

Getting the best results requires commitment. Not the sort of commitment needed to run an ultra-marathon but the kind to at least get out of bed each day, brush your teeth, and get dressed. These are the seemingly small commitments that become part of your habits and lifestyle. If you want your results to last long-term, you have to be committed to small changes long-term. This doesn't mean that you have to flip your life upside down. It simply means being committed to small changes—changes and adjustments to keep you in shape and feel good about yourself long term. "Commitment is one of the key ingredients for goal-success. If you're not fully committed to a goal, you won't give it all the effort required to succeed" (Roomer, 2019, para. 1). More often than not, we think that we are fully committed to our goals but then we begin to procrastinate and make bad decisions, which is a clear sign that we are not actually fully committed. In this case, you will fail to achieve your goals, not due to a lack of trying but due to a lack of commitment.

You may be relying on the initial motivation but are unable to sustain it. Commitment is something that becomes stronger with time. One way to develop a stronger commitment is to figure out why you have the desire in the first place. Why do you want to lose weight? Why do you want to eat healthier? Why do you want to make a change to your lifestyle? Once you have answered these questions in detail, your motivation will not be short lived.

When you have a strong sense of the reason behind your transformation, challenges won't throw you off so easily and it will be more difficult to give up. If you are uncertain of why you have chosen to undertake this journey, you would probably not step out of your comfort zone, you will be thrown off course more easily, and give up far quicker. If you know why you want to achieve your goals, you will be more likely to put in the necessary time and energy which will help lead you to success. You will be more disciplined and will defy all the odds by sticking to your routine.

A reminder that the first step to making these small changes is to write down the results you want and why you want them. Make a list to see what you want to achieve in black and white. The best place to start is to write down what you are currently not happy with and what results would make you happier than you are right now. You can write down anything you can think of relating not only to weight loss but also lifestyle, body shape, how you feel, and your eating habits. What's the point of writing down your goals? It will help you visualize what you want your future life to look like as well as your body shape, so you can be more committed. Each day will be easier to manage with this guided approach. Keep in mind that it is also important to reflect on your actions and steps, both successful and unsuccessful, to have an idea on how to improve it in the future. It will boost your confidence and motivation to act on what you have written down. In writing down your goals, it makes a better connection to your brain as the information is generally deemed as more of a 'confirmed fact' when something is written in black and white in front of you. It helps you to prioritize and steer yourself away from potential distractions. It is also essential to give yourself a deadline of sorts so that you can track and celebrate your progress. Without a deadline, there will be no target to focus on and you probably won't give it the seriousness that it deserves.

Try to picture how you will look in twelve weeks from now (this is the standard time for great body transformations). How do you look? How do you feel? What will have changed? How will you be balancing your weekly time to spend on your health and well-being? How much time will you be spending on other commitments? The answers to these questions will help you to plan your steps and shape the results you get by following my program. They will also help to make the necessary adjustments that will lead to lasting change. Some refer to this as Future Pacing which, "comes from a sport's psychology practice of visualizing success." (Williams, n.d., para. 1). So what this really means is that you imagine yourself in the future where you have already achieved the goal that you have set for yourself. More importantly, the pacing of this concept is related to the pace you will take to get where you want to be (yet again, realistic and at your own pace, not anyone else's), and what steps you are going to take to get there. With every successful step that you take as you are heading towards your goal, you see that it is possible to make improvements to your life, no matter how small they may be. Each small victory is one step closer towards your end goal—remember this, always!

Each person's results are unique to them. Everyone has a different body shape, a different lifestyle, different commitments, and different abilities. Never compare your progress to others! Your transformation is a journey which will be unique to you, and only you. By using Future Pacing techniques, it will help you focus on your own journey and not be thinking about others' progress, only your own.

# Chapter 7

# 80/20 Flexibility

*"My brother, Joe, started the Dolly Parton diet. It really made Joe lean Joe lean Joe lean Jooee lean."*

## Eating 80% Good Food and 20% Bad Food Is Realistic and Sustainable

I have created my own version of the 80/20 rule which can be applied to your eating habits. The original 80/20 rule is known as the Pareto Principle, whereby "80% of results will come from just 20% of the action" (Kruse, 2016, para. 4). My version is based on the balance between your intake of good food vs bad food (80% good, 20% bad). Personal nutrition can seem like a minefield; there are thousands, if not millions, of pages of information out there on food, nutrition, and weight loss. Most of this information will be useless to you when you follow my program as you only need to know a small amount of information for your unique needs. I will help you to identify the vital information needed for your own progress. I will help you to master your food intake to drastically improve your weight loss results. Eating healthy isn't just about losing weight, there are many long term, life improving benefits too.

According to *Medical News Today*, "A healthful diet typically includes nutrient-dense foods from all major food groups, including lean proteins, whole grains, healthful fats, and fruits and vegetables of many colors" (Crichton-Stuart, 2020, para. 1). Also, eating healthy can improve heart health, reduce the risk of cancer, improve your mood, improve gut health, improve your memory, assist with weight loss (one of our main focus points), assist with diabetes management, create strong bones and teeth, improve sleep, and improve the health of the next generation (especially if you have children of your own who will most likely follow most of your same eating habits).

When it comes to future generations, your children will follow your eating habits, so it is important to help them to create the 80/20 balance. How can you do this you may ask? If children eat with their families regularly (healthy meals that is), instead of with their friends, they will end up eating food with less sugar and healthier foods such as fruit and vegetables. Try to get your partner or your family at home on board with better meals too, it's always easier to eat well at home when you're all onboard with it. I've had client in the past that have felt demotivated and disheartened or even sometimes guilty because they're making healthier choices and their partners show little interest in their goals. Naturally, it isn't always doable to get everyone under your roof to sing from the same hymn sheets, but when your home life is a healthy one and it's deemed as normal, it will improve everyone's health not just yours. Be the leader, lead from the front and set a good example.

You don't need to follow a strict or fad diet, all you need to remember is to include each of the five main food groups in what you eat each day, and you will get all the nutrients you need. Let's look at the five major food groups: fruit and vegetables, carbs or starch, proteins, fats, and dairy. Do I have to eat five portions of fruit and vegetables a day? How am I going to get that right? This basically means that you will have to have either a fruit or vegetable with every meal, along with two snacks per day. My advice, is to start off with at least two good meals a day. Add fruit to your breakfast, and vegetables to dinner. It will just help to reduce your calorie intake and improve your digestion. Dairy is important for healthy teeth and bones as it contains a lot of calcium. On *Medicine Net*, there is great advice on how to divide your plate up so that you make sure you are getting in each of the five main food groups. They suggest doing the following:

"Vegetables fill half the plate, whereas proteins and grains fill the other half."

Most fad diets tell you to cut out carbs or starch completely, but it is vitally important not to do this as this is where most of your daily energy will come from, and the wholegrain versions also contain many vitamins and minerals (as surprising as that may seem). Meat, fish, and eggs contain the highest source of proteins and are all beneficial to heart health, better memory, good digestion, and, one of the main focal points (regarding appearance) for most women out there, protein promotes healthy skin and nails. Another food group that many diets recommend cutting out or making big reductions in is fat; however, there are some essential fats that your body needs to function optimally, and even reduce cholesterol, believe it or not. We need body fat and the consumption of various fat sources to give us energy, produce hormones and absorb certain vitamins. You cannot live without carbs, fat or protein if you want a basic level of good health.

Abstaining from eating specific food that you like will probably cause you to crave them even more. You might feel guilty if you eat the food you have cut out of your diet and feel like a failure because of it. You should continue to eat your favourite foods but just make sure to keep it to around 20% of your overall food intake. The reason I am so set on the 80/20 balance is because restrictive dieting could lead to overeating. When you try not to eat a certain food, that is all you end up thinking about. It could lead to awkward social situations because if your diet is restricted to such an extent, your choice of restaurants also becomes extremely limited, or you might completely avoid certain social situations so that you won't feel uncomfortable when you are the only one not ordering dessert. If you put too much unnecessary pressure on yourself, It may have an adverse effect on why you are doing all of this in the first place. The guilt of not following restrictive diets always becomes counterproductive, because guilt can lead to you giving up, and then you stop a diet and gain the weight back because their plan is too unsustainable, due to it being so restrictive.

## It Is Flexible and a Key Feature For Consistent Weight Loss

Approach your eating habits with flexibility and consistency and you are more likely to achieve consistent weight loss. You are going to have bad days, you are going to have good days, and you're going to have days when you feel guilty for eating a pizza or for having a few drinks and ordering take-out. This is completely normal. Anyone who gets great results and who eats healthy food consistently will tell you that you don't need to cut out your favourite food or treats all the time. To keep to the 80/20 balance, eating food that you enjoy is essential to creating healthy eating habits and for consistent weight management.

The first step to eating healthy is to eat nutrient-enriched food most of the time, not all of the time. To only ever eat nutrient-enriched food is almost impossible unless you want to stress yourself out so much that you end up failing. Most of my clients hit the ground running with this because you don't have to give up on eating treats, you are just adjusting the amount of good food you put into your body vs the crap you eat. Remember the balance; 80% good food and 20% bad food. I put together a Lean Food Guide which I give to all my clients and you can have access to it too, to jog your memory on good food. If you go to womenwhoconquer.co.uk/secretspdf you'll get my free How to Melt Your Love Handles guide and the Lean Food Guide PDF

The next step is to eat a relatively consistent amount of calories per day. You can monitor this with *MyFitness-Pal*; this is a free app to track your calorie intake by inputting the amount of pounds you want to lose per week and it will calculate your daily calorie intake for you. Don't worry about hitting the calorie goal or protein/carbohydrate or fat perfectly, you want to get as close as you can give or take about 20 grams on the macros. To give you body the proper intake of food it needs to function properly you must consume fat, carbs, and protein each day. Carbs are in foods like rice, pasta, bread, potatoes, and sugar. Protein is found in meat, fish, nuts, tofu, and eggs. Fats are found in eggs, meat, butter, cooking oils, cheese, and nuts.

Protein rich foods are extremely important for feeling fuller and satisfied for longer, and it also helps your body to burn fat as fuel. Protein will not give you big muscles. Most people do not consume enough protein, which leaves them feeling weaker and hungrier. Make sure that you are eating at least two fist-sized portions of meat or fish (or a protein alternative) as a general rule of thumb each day. There are a number of studies that show that the more protein you include in your diet, the better it will be for long-term weight loss and it will also increase the speed of your metabolism. It will also leave you feeling fuller for longer which will decrease your chances of wanting to have a quick, sugary and calorie-filled snack or meal. Thus, getting enough protein each day is hugely important for weight loss and burning calories. It is important at this point to bring in a few scientific facts, although this is not a scientific journal, this information is vital.

According to *Healthline*, there are ten science-backed reasons to eat more protein. These are: it reduces appetite and hunger levels, increases muscle mass and strength, promotes bone strength, reduces cravings and desire for late-night snacking, boosts metabolism and increases fat burning, lowers blood pressure, helps maintain weight loss, isn't harmful to healthy kidneys, helps the body repair itself after injury, and will help you to stay as fit as your age (Gunnars, 2019).

Thus, it can reduce your daily calorie intake for this reason. The easiest way to do this is to slightly reduce the amount of carbs and fats on your plate and slightly increase your protein portion. When exercising, no matter the intensity of it, it is important to increase your protein intake to help build and strengthen your muscles as well as speed up your recovery time after a workout session. It can also prevent losing muscle mass when losing weight.

If you are a vegetarian or a vegan, you must start paying close attention to your macros. A common issue that I've found with some of my clients over the years that are vegetarians or vegans, is that their protein levels are very low and both their carbohydrate and fat intake is higher than it should be, which means they tend to over eat and gain body fat. The main reason for this is the lack of protein, they feel more hungry and less satisfied from what they eat. The richest sources of protein are in meat and fish, so if you cut these out along with dairy and eggs, you'll have to find alternative sources of protein such as vegan protein powders, vegan friendly protein bars, nuts, tofu, Quorn and other alternative protein products. I guarantee that if your protein levels are low and you increase your protein intake to where it should be, you will notice a significant decrease in your hunger levels and you'll be able to excess body fat easier.

It is a myth that protein is bad for your bones. There is the common belief that the more protein you consume, the more acidic your body becomes, which is believed to use calcium from your bones to neutralize the acid. The truth is quite the opposite. This increase of protein in your diet is particularly important in order to keep your bones strong as you become older, especially for women who are more prone to osteoporosis as they age. Sometimes when you feel hungry, it is not because your body actually needs food and nutrients, it is just a craving for a certain taste or to feel good. How do you prevent this? It is simple, eat more protein, especially for breakfast. Consider that "a study in overweight adolescent girls found that eating a high-protein breakfast reduced cravings and late-night snacking" (Gunnars, 2019, para. 25). Eating more protein can also lower your blood pressure which, in the long run, can decrease your chances of having a heart attack or stroke for example.

By now we know that the more you increase your protein intake the less calories you will take in, and you will have less cravings and feel fuller for longer. You will see your weight start to fall, but in order to keep this weight off you will have to make extra protein a norm in your diet. Yet another myth is that an increase in protein in your diet will cause long-term harm to your kidneys. This is only the case for those with pre-existing kidney problems; for those with healthy kidneys, it will make no difference at all. If you have injured yourself, a protein-enriched diet can make your recovery time much shorter as protein helps to build up your body's tissues and organs, especially when we become older and our muscles begin to deteriorate. So eating more protein (and regular exercise) can not only prevent muscle loss as you age but also prevent your bones from becoming frail. Your calorie intake will never be perfect and neither will any of your other macros, it always fluctuates by a hundred or so calories, but the aim when you start out is to remain consistent. You want consistency, not perfection.

The quality of the majority of your food intake is important but it doesn't mean you have to eat everything organic or fresh, but we want as many vitamins and minerals from unprocessed food as possible. Vitamins and minerals are essential for 100's if not 1000's of processes inside the body. However, many foods aren't as rich in nutrients as they were 10-15 years ago, due to the quality of the soil we use to grow fruits and vegetables and anything food wise has been damaged due to heavy farming practices. So to be on the safe side, I recommend taking a good quality multi-vitamin and mineral supplement to top up your levels.

Avoid weight loss pills at all costs, they are not proven to work and there is no scientific evidence to prove it despite what reviews might say. They are generally high in caffeine which can cause you a whole host of issues even after a few days, such as heart palpitations, poor sleep and fatigue.

# Chapter 8

# Weight Loss Myths

*"I keep trying to lose weight, but it keeps finding me!"*

## Only Take Advice From Health or Weight Loss Professionals

I have heard some crazy weight loss hacks or tricks over the years and as you can imagine, they make me cringe. When it comes to maintaining weight loss, my advice is not to take any advice from diet, juicing or detox reps, not even friends, family or colleagues (unless of course they are health or weight loss professionals). More often than not, it is easier to take advice (that we will actually follow) from people we don't know as long as we see them as a professional in their area.

I am passionate about great results and I want to see the results that *last*. So when I overhear conversations about waist trainers or lemon juice for a breakfast "detox," or the classic "meal replacement juicing" diet, I get a little fired up. Why do I become so irate about these diets? It's because I know the process to weight loss is much simpler than people think and all the bad information and the false hope that these diets give do nothing but hold people back from achieving their ultimate goal.

I was lucky enough to have an article featured on FOX, CBS and NBC websites in the US; the headline was: "Diets are making you bigger, not slimmer." In this article, I spoke about the lasting damage that yo-yo diets can do to a woman's hormones and waistline. When your body undergoes prolonged periods of calorie restrictions or meal replacements (juicing), your body recognizes that it is not being fed properly and its defense mechanism is to store body fat. Why is this? It comes down to survival. Your body needs energy (food to survive and function), these kinds of diets put your body into what is basically survival mode. If you put your body through a phase of too much restriction, it will store fat in case you try to starve it again, resulting in starvation mode. This is your body's natural response to long-term calorie restriction. Your body will respond by storing those calories for energy to prevent actual starvation. When it comes to weight loss, this will never change, it will always depend on how many calories you take in vs how much you burn off with regular exercise. The aim is to burn more off than what you put in your mouth, coupled with regular exercise each week.

Are testosterone levels also important to note when trying to lose weight? Let's first talk about what testosterone is. It helps to develop and keep your muscle mass and strengthens your bones. This hormone seems to play a pretty important role when losing weight and keeping it off, especially for women who have reached menopause. If you don't have enough of this hormone, it can subsequently lead to weight gain—the very thing you are trying to avoid! So if you are not maintaining muscle as a result of low levels of testosterone, you are likely to eat more to make up for the loss of muscles. "Muscles burn far more calories than fat tissue. Lack of muscle thus puts people at a higher risk of eating too much and storing the excess calories as fat" (Arnarson, 2017, para. 15). The good news is that there is a way to help get a balance of this hormone in your body. If you want to do it the natural way, you can add some resistance training to your exercise regime, take in extra vitamin D and zinc, and make sure that you get a good night's rest each night because testosterone is produced mostly as we sleep to repair and recharge our bodies and maintain our muscle.

## Calories In vs Calories Out Remains the Most Important Principle for Weight Loss

The purpose of this chapter is to help you to get rid of any of the weight loss so-called theories out there, meaning all that nonsense about weight loss over the years. I am going to deconstruct the most common ones, as well as some of the crazy ones. There are seven particular myths that I feel you need to know about, to help understand how and why I chose to call my method of weight loss EASE.

The first myth claims that eating low fat or no fat will help you lose weight. Fat is absolutely essential for energy; it helps regulate your hormone production and helps your body take on certain vitamins from food. Your body can't function properly without it. Eating less fat or cutting it out completely will not help you lose weight and keep it off. Refer to MyFitnessPal for you daily fat intake.

The second myth claims that eating less carbs will help lose weight. Weight loss comes down to more calories being burnt each day than you eat. Your body needs carbs each day, mostly for energy and muscle repair, but eating less carbs doesn't necessarily mean you'll lose weight.

The third myth implies that some foods speed up your metabolism. There's no evidence that proves that any foods or supplements will speed up your metabolism. The only healthy way to speed up your metabolism and to help you burn more calories each day is to exercise more. If certain foods boost your metabolism, this would be the greatest discovery and they would be worth more than gold to many. The only healthy way to boost your metabolism is through exercise and good quality food to help keep your energy levels up. The combination of these two aspects helps your body recover and keeps your body working at its maximum capacity. A lack of exercise will slow your metabolism down, just as dieting or any kind of meal replacement or juicing will slow your metabolism down. When you starve the body it works at a slower rate to save energy and starts storing calories, hence why regularly skipping meals or yo-yo dieting isn't good for long term weight loss.

The fourth myth states that cardio workouts make you store fat. Everyone has to store fat around their muscles in order to recharge and protect your muscles. Cardio helps you to burn calories, not store them, as long as you're burning more calories than you consume.

The fifth myth claims that if the scales go up, you've gained body fat. Our weight fluctuates all day long. If you're losing weight and sometimes the scales show an increase in weight, it's highly likely that it's either extra water or food that makes it seem as though you have picked up weight. In order to gain one pound of body fat per week, you'd have to eat a minimum of 3500 extra calories per week. Remember, the scales aren't the only measurement tool to use that will keep track of your weight loss; you should also at least measure your waist and chest. This is because, as mentioned above, the scales might not go lower sometimes but you could still be burning body fat. When you reach your end goal, it will be how you look in the mirror in relation to how much body fat you've got rid of that will give you confidence, not just how many pounds you've lost. You might be 8lbs off your weight loss goal, but if you look great and you feel confident because you've seen such an amazing transformation with your body shape, the scales won't matter because you're 'in shape' vs being 'out of shape'.

The sixth myth is that if you skip meals, you'll lose more weight. One of the great things about eating breakfast, lunch and dinner is that it helps us to feel satisfied from the steady intake of nutrients throughout the day so that we don't get too hungry or tired. If you skip a meal, chances are that you're going to be extra hungry when you finally get the chance to eat, and the odds of wanting to grab quick, high sugar, high fat foods greatly increase. Skipping meals and binging at night time is a very common issue for people and often leads to fatigue, grumpiness and weight gain. I always advise my clients to eat a minimum of three times a day. You don't have to eat breakfast as soon as you get up but try and eat in the morning to get your energy flowing and keep the hunger at bay.

The last myth I would like to mention is the myth that lifting weights will give you big muscles. In order to build big muscles, the body needs to produce a lot of testosterone to do that. On average, men produce around

10-20 times more testosterone than women, which is why men typically have much more muscle mass than women. Lifting weights as a woman would not make you bulky because you generally don't have the testosterone to make big muscles like men do. When you see women on social media who have big solid muscles who are lifting weights and are clearly into bodybuilding, there's a good chance that they're taking some form of steroids or growth hormone in order to get big muscles. Lifting weights, even light weights, help to speed up your metabolism so you can burn more body fat without getting big muscles. The best case scenario is that you will have a more toned body shape.

If I lose weight too fast, will it slow down my metabolism? Yes, it most definitely can. Some diets force your body to break down your muscles to use as energy if you go to extremes like juicing, and once you have less muscle mass, your metabolism slows down. It is believed that certain types of foods can help to speed up your metabolism, but the easiest way to do this is to burn calories through exercise or simply reduce your calorie intake. This is the approach for yo-yo diets but as soon as you stop the diet or stop exercising, your muscle mass will decrease and your metabolism will slow down. It then becomes a lot easier to put body fat back on after coming off the diet. The three most effective forms of exercise that can help you to burn calories are aerobic activity (running, cycling, fitness classes and swimming), resistance training (lifting weights, body weight exercises, as muscles burn more calories than fat), or being active in some way or the other (like taking a long walk).

When it comes to calories, there are some foods that are believed to be unhealthy but are actually not. Potatoes, bread and pasta, for example, may seem bad but it is just because they can be used for a variety of different dishes which makes it easy to eat too much of them. Try to balance the types of foods on your plate with extra veggies and protein. Breakfast cereal is also another food that might be seen as unhealthy, yet some are packed with vital nutrients like iron and vitamin B. Whole wheat and not gluten-free foods are also good for the health of your gut. You may have heard that bananas have far more sugar than most fruits but they are an excellent source of potassium, vitamin C (which we commonly associate with citrus), and fibre.

# Chapter 9

# Creating Your Plan

*"Everyone has a plan, until they get punched in the face."*

— MIKE TYSON

## Having a Plan Will Give You Clarity

Sometimes (actually a lot of the time) life gets in the way of our plans. That is why it is important to have a solid plan with definite steps to follow so that you ensure a successful outcome when following my program. Having a solid plan will help you to have a guide to get back on track if life throws you off course. Remember that an idea without a plan is just a dream. It is also best to plan for all possible outcomes, knowing that life hardly ever goes 100% according to plan. In our case, how would we plan for all possible outcomes? Firstly, you may need to extend your timeline if you don't meet your goal in the designated time that you give yourself because you won't know how much weight you can realistically lose until you actually start losing weight and tracking it once a week. Secondly, all outcomes could also refer to an unavoidable obstacle that you might need to face, like getting the flu or having a family emergency. The main idea here is that no matter what the plan is, it is always important to have one. Be flexible with the plans you make and become willing to make adjustments (if necessary) as you go along. Take time to plan properly, don't just spend a few minutes on your plan and expect it to be failproof. At the beginning of your journey, your plan may seem perfect but we all learn as we go along, so be adaptable in your approach. You should always have a plan B, like adjusting your exercise days/times or pre planning what you might do for lunch if you're travelling for work, in this way, "you'll be ready to face anything with the right mixture of preparedness and flexibility" (Russo, 2015, para. 14). Sometimes plan B ends up turning out much better than plan A as you might have had to work harder for it. Thus, the reward will be greater in the end.

There is a solution to most things that you want to change in your life, but it does require thoughtful planning. We are able to gain emotional stability through making plans as we realize that there is a solution and steps that we can take to make our lives better. The main purpose of having a plan is to have an objective that you are heading towards, but this does not mean that it will turn out perfectly. Without a sure plan for your weight loss goals, it will be like putting all your energy into something that will have no positive results, like pouring water into a bucket full of holes. These goals could give you a sense of purpose, being excited to wake up in the morning, and it won't really seem like hard work if you want it enough. Twelve weeks seems long at first, but once you get started with my program, it will pass by faster than you thought it could. I don't want to call them deadlines, but I do want to add that your plan should have a time frame (you should have a plan for each week of the program and adjust it as you progress). I am pretty sure that most people agree that the more prepared you are before starting something, the more confident you will be to stay the course, and because you have back up plans, you can always move on to any of them if you feel the first one is not working. This allows you to keep the momentum going. It might even motivate you to take risks because you know that you have alternate plans to fall back onto.

This step is a fun one, well I find it fun anyway, and I'm sure you will enjoy it too. This is where you get to map out your plan to reach your end goal as quickly and as realistically as possible. Each time I coach a client, one of the first things we do is map out a personalized plan for them. We do this together on a call as it is important that each of my clients understands exactly how they are going to get to where they want to be, and exactly what they are going to do to get there. A plan doesn't need to be pages and pages full of countless goals, it just needs to be a few bullet points for your weekly goals and then what your long-term goals I do believe that it is important to always have a plan B though. As previously discussed, things go wrong all the time, life gets in the way, motivation dwindles, and commitment is not constant. By having a plan B, you are giving yourself the potential to prevent failure before it happens. When you begin to change your old habits, add this one to your list. "Just like fastening your seat belt, using a plan B approach can and should become habit-forming" (Bush, 2012, para. 5). You can seamlessly change your course of action if you see that your current one is not working.

The first step is to list your goals. Realistically, how much weight do you want to lose? How many dress sizes would you like to drop? Weight is important to measure in your plan but it is certainly not the only aspect that you need to focus on in order for you to transform your body. Remember, you are not aiming for perfection or to completely overhaul your lifestyle. You are looking to make small changes, one step at a time.

You will need to measure your weight, waist and chest and monitor these measurements once a week. It is ideal to make these measurements at the beginning of the week and first thing in the morning and not on a Saturday morning after a few glasses of wine and having pizza the night before. Another important step to monitor your progress is to take pictures of yourself (I know that most of you will feel uneasy about taking these but it is important to use these) so you can see the physical transformation from the moment you start the program until you have reached your goal. I ask my client to take these pictures about 4 weeks apart as you should see a distinct difference after each month of following your plan. By looking at the pictures you have taken, it will show you how much progress you have made and motivate you to continue with your plan of action and see what a difference these changes have made to your health. Think about the times you have seen other women's before and after pictures and thought, "Wow! She looks great now, tons better than before. What an amazing difference!" Even though you might want to keep your pictures private, they become another great motivator to reach your goal.

## Keep Your Plan Simple and Realistic

Keep your plan simple so that you won't feel intimidated by it and shy away from it from the get-go. It will make you feel that it is possible to achieve and not something that only an Olympic athlete will be able to do. We will look at the changes you need to make to your eating habits to help you reach your goals. Maybe you need to drink more water each day, drink less alcohol, or order less take-out. Buy food at the start of each week and eat at least two decent meals per week, instead of grabbing food on the go, which is generally unhealthy food. Also, you need to avoid skipping meals so that your body does not go into survival mode and start to store fat. Healthy food does not have to be fancy; stick to simple, easy to make meals, and eat the healthy food that you actually enjoy. I don't know about you but any meal with kale in it is certainly not a *tasty* healthy meal. Remember the 80/20 rule, eat 80% good food and around 20% bad food within each week to be realistic and make your eating habits sustainable, long term.

We will also look at how much exercise you can realistically fit in each week. To lose weight effectively and keep it off, you don't need to start off with intense workouts. It could simply mean taking a walk a few times a week or making sure that you walk a little farther each day, all while going about your regular schedule. If you have workout equipment at home, it could mean using that a few times a week. With your exercise routine, just like eating healthy food that you like, do the exercise that you like the most, whether it be walking, running, cycling, swimming, or whatever else you may enjoy. I set these exercise goals with each client as their abilities differ and some prefer certain types of exercise over others. Start with short workouts (around fifteen minutes) three times a week, and increase the time that you exercise every few weeks. My clients also have access to twelve weeks worth of short, home workout videos that don't require any equipment to complete.

When it comes to exercise, always work according to your own abilities and remember what I said in the beginning of the book: Start where you are. If that means walking three times a week, or for a short time every day, then that is where you start. Do not start with a high intensity 30 minute CrossFit session. That will defeat the purpose of slowly increasing the time spent on exercise as well as the intensity of it. Even if the only exercise that you do is taking your dog for longer walks a few times a week, that is a great start! Remember that getting started is the most important part and keeping it as a regular part of your week is just as important to build a habit out of it; you can build on that as you progress in your program.

Another important factor to keep in mind is to learn to be flexible with your plan. Should life punch you in the face and you need to change the days or time of day that you exercise, then it is okay to change it. Be open to change as you go along, so that you don't become totally unmotivated and beat yourself up about skipping your regular Tuesday afternoon walk, or whatever exercise you are doing at that stage. With the food that you eat, if you get bored with eating the same meals, then try out some new ones. Have a flexible approach to your plans. This always works the best as life throws us many curve balls, there will always be changes taking place, so we need to be able to adapt to change. The ones who get great results are the ones who continue to eat well and exercise regularly in spite of the changes taking place in their lives.

So let's breakdown your weekly goals:

**No.1** - Track your food with MyFitnessPal every single day, with a realistic 80% good food and 20% bad food approach (make sure you set the app to lose 2lbs/1kg per week). It's a numbers game, the numbers don't lie, and what's measurable is manageable. Guess work is one of the reasons people on diets struggle to understand what their needs are food wise, because you're basically guessing that if you eat less of certain foods you can keep the weight off and hit your ultimate weight loss goal. Diets do not give you specific data about your personal food intake needs, MyFitnessPal does which is why myself and thousands of coaches worldwide use it, because it works.

The goal is not to be in a calorie deficit forever, only till you reach your weight loss or body shape goal, so then you can increase your calories by a few hundred each day.

**No.2** - Start moving more every day. Tracking your steps is a great place to start for the first few weeks (aiming for 10k steps) but you don't want to become reliant on walking alone as some people can easily get used to it and it can be difficult to shift body fat at a decent pace. The best way to speed up your metabolism and burn a good amount of calories in a short space of time is to do short workouts. Some beginner workout videos (no equipment needed) as short as 15 minutes are fantastic for toning up and burning body fat, which is what most of my clients have used for the past 5-6 years.

Aim for 2 – 3 short workouts per week, then every 3 – 4 weeks you can either go up to 20 – 30 minute workouts 3 times a week or follow some 15 minute workouts 3-4 times per week. It all comes down to what workouts are going to fit into your schedule best, and short workouts are perfect for developing flexible exercise habits and getting leaner.

You have to increase what you do as you get fitter and stronger, to keep your metabolism high so you can burn the maximum calories possible each day. You might get into fitness classes or jogging or other forms of exercise, which is great, you should also aim to do exercise that you actually enjoy and not just to lose weight because to keep the results long term, exercise must be part of your lifestyle.

**No. 3** – Tracking your weight once a week, on the same day, first thing in the morning after you've been to the toilet and before you drink or eat anything, measuring your weight in the morning will give you a true reading on your weight loss. Your weight fluctuates throughout the day and throughout the week, that's why we measure it once a week so you don't get confused when your body is 2-3 pounds heavier at 6pm compared to 6am from all the food and water, make sense? Keep a record of your weight loss somewhere too.

They are your bread-and-butter goals each week. How you exercise and when you exercise is entirely up to you, what time of the day you track your food is entirely up to you too, it's your lifestyle at the end of the day so you should be aiming to build exercise into your schedule in small blocks along with food tracking. Write down in a planner or a diary your exercise schedule each week to help you stay on track and make adjustments if needed.

# Chapter 10

# Motivation, Stress and Building Habits

*"People say nothing is impossible, but I do nothing every day."*

— *WINNIE THE POOH*

## Motivation Is Not Enough, You Must Create Habits

If you want long term results, you must create habits that become part of your everyday life. Motivation always fluctuates and can be nonexistent some days. Have you ever woken up one morning and thought, "Fuck it! I'm not going to do any exercise or do anything constructive today, in fact, I'm just going to binge watch Netflix and eat a whole lot of junk food." Sometimes we have to push ourselves through our excuses and through our laziness, even when motivation is low. Now I know that this is always easier said than done but we need to accept the fact that we are not always going to be able to operate at full capacity every single day—we are human, not machines. I need to accept that I'm not always going to be motivated; I'm not always going to do everything I need to each day and, most importantly, my motivation is going to fluctuate from day to day. But don't give up! Consistency each week is what we're looking for, so we can afford to have those days where we don't eat as well or exercise because we're not motivated enough, be flexible with your motivation as you are with your eating habits.

When you visualize yourself looking slimmer, wearing nice clothes, feeling confident and living a healthy lifestyle, that will be because you kept going even when you didn't have the motivation some days. This is because you built the habit and did it regardless of whether you had a fight with your partner or had a bad week. Our motivation is not a constant; it fluctuates daily. Some days we are excited but other days we couldn't care less. It's our habits that keep us going, and keep everything in our lives in check. We get out of bed and brush our teeth out of habit, and we do it regardless of what mood we are in. We drive our cars like we are on autopilot because we don't have to think much about how to drive anymore. We build habits and the awareness of them just as we develop the habit of driving a car. At first, we have to consciously think about and be aware of each step but after a while it becomes second nature and we do it regardless of our levels of motivation or how we feel.

When first developing a new habit or curbing an old one, it is imperative that you don't try to change your whole lifestyle at once. If you try to do too much too soon, you are destined to fail. There are three basic things that make up habits (Ferebee, 2018). The first is what triggers you to follow the normal course of action out of habit or survival mode, based on how you feel, or the environment surrounding you that triggers certain habitual reactions. The second is the actual action that you take. Keep doing it if it's benefiting you, but if not then it's time to break the habit and replace it with one that is constructive. Thirdly, when developing a new, positive habit, you will feel a sense of accomplishment when you get it right. This can motivate you to keep doing the same action so that you can feel good about yourself, including boosting your self-esteem and self-confidence. Some habits are easier to continue than others as you get an instant reward for putting in very little effort. For example, drinking alcohol or smoking to relax; the alcohol or nicotine gives you an instant rush of dopamine which motivates you to continue as the output is greater than the input. You will be less motivated to continue positive behavior if you don't see an instant change or receive instant gratification, making it more difficult to make long lasting changes to your habits. You know that it will be good for you in the long run, but are you willing to stick it out and stay the course to get the eventual reward? If you do manage to stick it out, the reward will be far more gratifying, as the saying goes, "anything of value takes time to achieve."

Make it easier for yourself by exercising where you feel the most comfortable and not spending hours at the gym or paying for a gym membership that you hardly ever make use of. Don't have a crazy amount of goals that you are so eager to achieve but the timeframe in which you want to achieve it is totally unrealistic. Set small goals for yourself each day and once you achieve these small goals, you will develop a good habit, feel good about yourself, and begin to set more of these goals or a bit more challenging goals. Exercising regularly and eating well can become a habit, just as I have illustrated with my previous example of driving. Yes, it takes time and effort but it is possible to make them part of your lifestyle. Remember that it will take time to create the life you want through changing your habits. Of course, motivation is great and it helps a lot. It can sometimes be the spark you need to get started on something, but it rarely lasts too long. We build habits by taking repeated action, with or without motivation. This is sometimes hard to do, but that's when you can push through and develop much stronger habits by doing them repeatedly, even when you are not in the mood to do anything. Change is stressful. Remember this going in, if we embrace change, it will make us even stronger in the process. Our potential to embrace change is not only related to adversities but can also be applied to exercise regime and improve our performance and progress.

According to *Mindfulness Muse*, there are three C's related to how we approach stress; this stands for Committed, Control, and Challenge (Schenck, n.d.). If you are *Committed* enough to your journey, you will stay the course. You should remain diligent in following your goals, meaning giving it your absolute best effort. People who are strong in *Control* will have the attitude that no matter how difficult things may get, they will not succumb to the stress. We cannot necessarily change our circumstances or the actions of others, but we can change our own thoughts and how we approach anything in life. We can either see adversity as having the potential to stop us in our tracks, or we can see it as an opportunity to learn something instead of becoming so stressed out that we begin to feel powerless. Strong people see stress as a norm and see it as a potential to grow. These people see stressful situations as a *Challenge* instead of a threat and see it from an optimistic perspective. It is inevitable that change is going to cause some degree of stress.

## Take Regular Time Out to Reduce Stress Levels

Taking regular time for yourself ("me time") is important for your physical and psychological well-being, it may lead to psychological problems if you focus on and put too much time into work and don't make enough time to take a breather. Stress is a silent killer. It can kill your desire to eat well; it can kill your exercise routine; it can kill your energy levels. When we experience stress, we might stop looking after ourselves properly because it can make us feel physically and mentally exhausted. It can change the way we behave, not just to ourselves and our health, but towards others too, which can have an overall negative impact on our lives. Stress and a high workload can often lead to skipping meals, craving food with a high sugar or fat content, and drinking more alcohol. It is important to be aware of your stressors, the triggers that cause stress, and what is causing you stress at the present moment and try to reduce it as much as possible.

One of the best ways to take time out for yourself is to do some exercise to relieve some stress and take your mind off what is stressing you out. Exercise can make you feel good about yourself (by releasing those endorphins) and it is obviously good for your physical well-being too (by lowering your blood pressure after your workout). Do some form of exercise that you enjoy, whether it be a walk outside in the fresh forest air, a run around the block, pilates, yoga, or anything else that you prefer. There are also other ways to perform self-care, something that will help you reduce stress and completely switch off, whether it be gardening or painting or getting your hair done. It could serve as a creative outlet or a chance to socialize with new people. Go for a massage or treat yourself to a facial or go get your nails done. Pampering yourself will definitely make you feel more relaxed afterwards. Have a nap and make sure to have a good laugh—do whatever it takes to relieve some stress. Taking time out of your schedule for yourself is how you can nurture yourself and have the physical and mental capacity to deal with what life throws your way.

Identification of stress is important, so that you can deal with it better and know what your starting point is. According to the *Mental Health Foundation*, these are the common signs that help us to identify stress ("How to Manage and Reduce Stress," n.d.):

- Feelings of constant worry or anxiety
- Feelings of being overwhelmed
- Difficulty concentrating
- Mood swings or changes in your mood
- Irritability or having a short temper
- Difficulty relaxing
- Depression
- Low self-esteem
- Eating more or less than usual
- Changes in your sleeping habits

- Substance abuse
- Aches and pains, particularly muscle tension
- Diarrhoea or constipation
- Nausea or dizziness
- Loss of sex drive

If you are experiencing one or more of the above symptoms, it is likely that you are stressed. Once you have identified this, it is easier to come up with a plan to combat the stress (or just lessen) in your everyday life. You can also attempt to identify the origins or causes so that you can do something to change it and reduce the amount of stress in your life. Then it is time for a reality check! Take an honest look at your lifestyle and think about what changes you could make to prevent excess stress in the first place.

Exercise and eating well has proven to help reduce stress and release tension from our bodies, both physically and mentally. If you remember to eat regularly and exercise it will not only help you feel better, but it will help you manage your stress better. Exercise builds mental resilience as you're pushing yourself through the exercises to see it through to the end, so repeated workouts each week allows your body to handle physical and psychological stress better. However, this is not the only way to manage stress. Have as much "me time" as possible and do it several times a day if this is viable for you in your busy schedule—even if it's just for ten minutes. It can help you relax and recharge just enough to feel a bit better and stay focused. You are the owner of your own lifestyle, it's up to you to take breaks and take care of yourself. Take ownership of health and ways to improve it (physically, emotionally, and mentally) as it will not only reduce stress, it will make you feel confident, healthy, happy, and motivated.

Here are seven steps according to the *Mental Health Foundation* that will serve as a reminder of and summary of how to protect yourself from stress ("How to Manage and Reduce Stress," n.d.):

1. Develop healthy eating habits.

2. Try to minimize smoking and you reduce your alcohol intake, or even cut it out completely.

3. Do regular exercise.

4. Remember to take time out for yourself and don't forget to incorporate self-care into your everyday habits.

5. Pay attention to how you feel and what you think in certain situations so that you will be able to better manage stressful situations and make better choices.

6. Make sure you get enough sleep.

7. Remember that one day of failure to follow a good habit does not make you or your entire life a failure.

# Chapter 11

# How To Tenaciously Face Adversity

*"Start by doing what's necessary; then do what's possible; and suddenly you are doing the impossible."*

— FRANCIS OF ASSISI

## Obstacles Are Inevitable

When you are trying to make a change to your lifestyle, especially changes in your usual habits, it is sure to be challenging sometimes. Especially when changing a diet that you have been following for years or an exercise regime (even if it is not working optimally), it will always be difficult to replace old habits with new, constructive ones. It is vitally important to look after your health and change your lifestyle choices to ones that are more conducive to healthy living. Take heart and have courage to face these adversities and, most importantly, don't allow this to discard your plans altogether!

How do you do this? The first thing you need to do is build a stable support system, to hold you accountable but also, if things go awry, you have one or a few go-to people who can help you get back on your feet. "Look for people who believe in you and your vision. Surround yourself with the people who will encourage you and help you have the strength and determination to keep going" (Murray, 2017, para. 8). We all need a cheerleader in our lives to tell us to keep going, that everything will turn out okay in the end, and be there when things are on their way to falling apart. These people could also help you regain your motivation to keep going in spite of what others think or say. They'll help keep you on your feet no matter what life throws at you.

Try not to focus on your negative thoughts as this could develop into a vicious cycle that will be difficult to break. Learn from what is not working and try other options. There's no point in being stuck in a rut. If you feel that your weight has plateaued and you're unhappy with it, then there is no point in carrying on with the same exercises that you have been doing for months. Don't panic! Remember earlier in the book where I mentioned that you should have a backup plan? Move swiftly to this option to keep the momentum going.

If you are finding it difficult to keep to the 80/20 food (calorie) intake, try new healthy food or new recipes; the chances are that you are simply bored with the food that you have been eating for months on end. Also, don't carry the burden of your failures along with you into your future, this serves no valuable purpose. Only carry the lessons that you have learnt along the way. Sometimes obstacles can overwhelm and destabilize us so that we will no longer be able to focus on our original plan. Focus on your small victories as these will inevitably lead to your desired outcome. Progress is progress, no matter how small it may seem to you. Remember to give yourself a pat on the back for each accomplishment. This will help you move forward. Reflect on and re-evaluate your goals if you are feeling stuck; a tweak here and there could make the world of difference. Have courage to keep on track, even if external factors threaten your new and healthier lifestyle.

Here are some tips to consider when facing adversity in your weight loss journey: Have faith in yourself—your state of mind is more important than the situation because that is where courage, strength, and miracles are born. Develop positive inner dialogue like, "I can do this," rather than, "I am a failure. I might as well quit now." Know you have nothing to lose. If you have true faith in yourself, the only loss you will experience will be worry, fear, and things you cannot control. Remember, this isn't the end, as challenges will always be a part of life, so the quicker you learn a method to cope with and overcome these challenges, the better it will be for you in the long run. Use it to cultivate a stronger version of yourself and a more solid ability to never give up (Scott, 2021).

Think of adversity as something positive as we can learn a great deal from it and it builds confidence, character, and resilience. If we feel defeated, it is difficult to deal with the present challenges we face. Learning to deal with adversity is an absolutely necessary tool to think more clearly about what we are facing, in order to deal with it more constructively. It will also give us more confidence to face and deal with obstacles we may face in the future. It is pointless to resist it, otherwise it will stifle your growth and leave you miserable enough to throw a pity party. Let's be totally honest for a moment though. None of us welcome adversity or obstacles in our lives; however, we should expect that we will constantly come across them. Thus, it is better to learn how to deal with and overcome them, so that it becomes easier the next time we are faced with it. We might not know exactly how to deal with what life throws our way at first but we will at least have a starting point and some resources to draw from when needed. Have "faith that everything will work out; faith that there is always light at the end of the tunnel, and faith that 'this too shall pass.' Everything in life has its place and purpose" (Hereford, n.d., para. 12).

How do we build up resilience though? As Nietzsche said, "what does not kill me makes me stronger" (1990, p. 2). This is not always the case as if you don't know how to adequately deal with adversity, it can derail your plans and put you off attempting to meet that goal again. Your resilience will strengthen as you go along and the more obstacles you face, the more adept you will become at handling them. For example, you are one week into your weight loss program and your car breaks down; it will cost a lot to fix but you don't necessarily have cash at hand to fix it. How will you get to work now? If you live close enough to work, why not change your plan a little and walk to work, instead of adding your exercise time to later in the day? Now I'm not saying that you should walk through a blizzard, you can always order an Uber, but what I am saying is that you need to learn to improvise. Another example is if you are used to walking your dog a few times a week but they get sick, you could always haul out that bicycle that has been collecting dust for many years and cycle around the block a few times. The important point here is that you need to remain flexible throughout the duration of your program and beyond. You could also "take inspiration and learn from others who have dealt successfully with adversity" (Hereford, n.d., para. 16). Life is never predictable so we need to be creative in coming up with solutions for the roadblocks that we are bound to face, especially when implementing change into our daily routine.

## Don't Let Any Adversity Throw You Off Course

It is all about how you approach what life throws at you and how you handle it. Do you see it as an opportunity for growth or as something that will completely throw you off course? "Adversity can feel like an uphill battle, especially when you're not getting a break from it. However, successful people have found a way to navigate their way around roadblocks that would stop others in their tracks" (Elizabeth, 2020, para. 4). If you resist adversity, you will only make it more difficult for yourself, so, instead, just go with it and deal with it one small step at a time, just like the planning process and execution of your weight loss regime. Learn to have self-compassion, and by this I don't mean feeling sorry for yourself but going easy on yourself. Sometimes it is easier to be compassionate towards others than towards yourself, but you still need to remember that you have everything you need to navigate through any hardships.

Learn to control your emotions because the way you approach obstacles will determine whether or not you successfully overcome them. If you are feeling negative, there is no need to allow these thoughts to consume you and the way that you behave. Try to find humor in the situation. I don't mean avoid it and pretend it is not there but some comic relief will help to relieve some of the stress. Use those positive emotions to your advantage. With this as your starting point, you will be placed on better footing than if you saw it as all doom and gloom. It will also help you to be more rational when trying to come up with a solution for the problem. Anything that alleviates your mood, makes you happier and feel more inspired will give you hope no matter what the negative external factors might be. It will also serve you well to not ask questions such as, "Why is this happening to me?" or "Why do bad things always happen to me?" If you remain positive, you might be able to figure out why you are being faced with this so-called bad luck and rise above the situation. "You may be surprised by how much calmer you feel in the face of adversity when you choose to find strength and joy during the darkest of times" (Elizabeth, 2020, para. 24). Lastly, you need to believe in yourself just enough to think beyond the present moment and not see it as the end of the world. How you approach adversity will determine whether or not you will overcome it, and you will experience personal growth if you do. The more adversities you overcome, the more confident you will be when facing future adversities as you can look back and think, "If I could overcome this or that, I will certainly be able to overcome this too!"

In essence, don't allow adversity to overwhelm you, be adaptable, keep your eye on the prize, don't allow others to be a source of discouragement, and stay the course, no matter what!

# Conclusion

## Success Stories

I have helped hundreds of women reach their weight loss goals and I can't wait to help thousands more. It will definitely not be instant gratification but it certainly will be worth it at the end of the twelve weeks. It doesn't stop there though! It's long-term and as long as you stick to the plan and the formula, you will be able to keep off the weight you have lost. Just a reminder of the EASE method from Chapter 5 (Evaluation and aims, Accountability and support, Simple to understand, and Easy to implement), it really does work. Here are a few testimonies of success stories from my clients to show you that you, too, can be successful (see my website – http://www.womenwhoconquer.co.uk for video interviews and transformation pictures):

"I now feel so much more positive mentally and way more energetic. I have been able to do 4 home workouts as well as participating in hockey and tennis while sticking to my calorie intake (even with a few treats) and I have lost weight!!!"

"I have lost 4.4 pounds in the last week which is crazy for me as my weight has not dropped in about 2 or 3 years despite my activity levels so Adam must know what he is talking about as this is basically a miracle!"

"I was worried when we first started our journey that I wouldn't lose any weight but gain muscle (as I have in the past), but after 3 months and 10 kilos lost (22lbs, which have stayed off and I've lost more) I've learnt to eat right but not cut out anything. Still really appreciative of what you help me achieve Adam"

"I feel like I've got my confidence back. I feel so much better than I did twelve weeks ago!! My body shape has changed so much and it shows on the scales as well. And for other people to keep saying to me that I look good makes me want to carry on!

I know, yeah, last year I had put weight on not lost it! And I was paying a PT. I honestly can't believe how far I've come in just 12 weeks it's amazing. That's why I came back to you, I knew you'd get me results"

"10 weeks in total with Adam Grayston, 17.8lb lost, 3.5 inches off my chest, 3.35 off my waist, 3 inches off my hips and 7.6lbs off my 3$^{rd}$ stage goal"

(Women Who Conquer, n.d.)

"Grayston helps women to banish diets for good with his innovative blueprint for success" ( "Transformation Coach Adam Graystom to Women Around the World," 2021).

I have a free 'Melt Your Love Handles Secrets' pdf which is available for download from my website: http://www.womenwhoconquer.co.uk/secretspdf. It contains my top eight tips for shifting that first 2-4 pounds of body fat.

## The Formula Is Really Simple

According to my research and experience, most women don't realize that their bodies' reaction or defense mechanism against diets and prolonged calorie restriction leads to weight gain. This research indicates that if the body isn't being fed enough food, or if meals are being skipped regularly, it will actually start to store fat and ultimately lead to more weight gain. Calories in vs calories out and regular exercise is a proven formula that has never changed. It doesn't matter how many pills, trends, or diets you try, our biology is designed to lose weight and keep it off with this formula. The skill (or art, as I prefer to view it) is combining it all together to make it as effective as possible for you. No matter how many times someone tries to reinvent the wheel when it comes to weight loss, the simple foundation of it is calories in vs calories out. Many people just find some unsustainable diet to play around with for quick results until it backfires and they can't sustain that method anymore, then the weight starts to creep back up. Don't reinvent the wheel—go with what works!

These crash diets will damage your body in the long run, no one (by choice) should feel the need to starve themselves or restrict their diet to such an extent that meals are no longer enjoyed. You may even become so strict with a diet that it could affect your work or your relationships. If you have children, they are meant to discover and decide which foods they enjoy and the ones they don't. If your diet restricts the variety of their food intake, you could be damaging their healthy growth and cause them to have a bad relationship with food. It is clear that crash diets don't only negatively affect you physically but mentally too. You will end up feeling like a failure just because you might have eaten one extra biscuit than you should have; this is most definitely not a healthy thought pattern.

While this isn't great news for chronic dieters, the good news is that most damage done by diets can be reversed. You can get back down to a healthier, happier weight with more confidence and rebalance your hormonal response to food. You just need to be open minded and willing to change your preconceived ideas about your eating habits and diets with these new tools in this book. Now that you know that there is an alternative, will you take the first step? You can do this! You will get results, reaching your goals is possible, and you do have what it takes for you to accomplish them. You have read enough success stories to know that this is certainly far from a hoax and it is possible for anyone to achieve. The choice is yours.

Now that you have all the tools, go out there and use them to become the best version of yourself. If you enjoyed the book, please leave a review on Amazon.

# References

Abbate, E. (2017, October 24). "Why you should give up restrictive dieting once and for all." Shape. https://www.shape.com/weight loss/tips-plans/why-you-should-stop-restrictive-dieting

Ackerman, C. (2021, March 22). "Writing therapy: Using a pen and paper to enhance personal growth." Positive Psychology. https://positivepsychology.com/writing-therapy/

Acton, A. (2017, November 3). "How to set goals (and why you should write them down)." Forbes. https://www.forbes.com/sites/annabelacton/2017/11/03/how-to-set-goals-and-why-you-should-do-it/?sh=6783de4e162d

Andrews, R. (2021). "18 ways to start transforming your body immediately." Precision Nutrition. https://www.precisionnutrition.com/18-ways-to-transform-your-body

Arnarson, A. (2017, July 18). "Can boosting your testosterone help you lose fat?" Healthline. https://www.healthline.com/nutrition/testosterone-and-fat-loss

Ashe, A. (2015, January 7). "Start where you are. Use what you have. Do what you can." Oncology Nursing News. https://www.oncnursingnews.com/view/start-where-you-are-use-what-you-have-do-what-you-can

Beale, M. (2020, July 20). "Future pacing | Top NLP technique." NLP Techniques. https://www.nlp-techniques.org/future-pacing/

Bush, S. (2012). "Always have a plan b." Tough Nickel. https://toughnickel.com/business/always-have-a-plan-b

CABA With You For Life. (n.d.). "Taking time out for yourself." https://www.caba.org.uk/help-and-guides/information/taking-time-out-yourself

Cassetty, S. (2019, November 26). "5 seemingly unhealthy foods that are actually good for you." NBC News Better by Today. https://www.nbcnews.com/better/lifestyle/5-seemingly-unhealthy-foods-are-actually-good-you-ncna1090926

Choi, J. (2020, December 17). "Stepping stones will get you to your destination." Life Hack. https://www.lifehack.org/642026/642026

Clear, J. (2018, October 16). "Forget about setting goals. Focus on this instead." James Clear. https://james-clear.com/goals-systems

Crichton-Stuart, C. (2020, December 10). "What are the benefits of eating healthy?" Medical News Today. https://www.medicalnewstoday.com/articles/322268

Economy, P. (2018, February 28). "This is the way you need to write down your goals for faster success." Inc. https://www.inc.com/peter-economy/this-is-way-you-need-to-write-down-your-goals-for-faster-success.html

Edberg, H. (2021, February 24). "How to take action: Twelve habits that turn dreams into reality." The Positivity Blog. https://www.positivityblog.com/how-to-take-action/

Elizabeth, A, (2020, December 4). "5 powerful tips for overcoming adversity." Life Hack. https://www.lifehack.org/866219/overcoming-adversity

Ferebee, A. (2018, February 13). "The science behind adopting new habits (and making them stick)." Forbes https://www.forbes.com/sites/quora/2018/02/13/the-science-behind-adopting-new-habits-and-making-them-stick/?sh=2895f88a43c7

Ferrari, J. (2010). "Psychology of procrastination: Why people put off important tasks until the last minute." American Psychological Association. https://www.apa.org/news/press/releases/2010/04/procrastination

Finkelstein, D. (n.d.). "Why is being accountable so important?" Tick Those Boxes. https://tickthoseboxes.com.au/why-is-being-accountable-so-important/

Flaherty, R. (2019, June 4). "The five 'hidden' reasons that stopped me losing weight." The Irish Times. https://www.irishtimes.com/life-and-style/health-family/fitness/the-five-hidden-reasons-that-stopped-me-losing-weight-1.3907044

"Golden rules of goal setting." (n.d.) Mind Tools. https://www.mindtools.com/pages/article/newHTE_90.htm

Grayston, A. (2021, March 31). "Adam Grayston - Body transformation coach." Local Gyms and Fitness. https://www.localgymsandfitness.com/GB/Longridge/2439382657326twelve/Adam-Grayston---Body-Transformation-Coach

Guise, S. (n.d.). "3 reasons to always have a plan." Stephen Guise. https://stephenguise.com/3-reasons-to-always-have-a-plan/

Gunnars, K. (2019, March 8). "10 science-backed reasons to eat more protein." Healthline. https://www.healthline.com/nutrition/10-reasons-to-eat-more-protein

Gunnars, K. (2019, October 2). "Is 'starvation mode' real or imaginary? A critical look." Healthline. https://www.healthline.com/nutrition/starvation-mode

Hazlewood, T. (2018, July 4). "Start where you are, use what you have, do what you can." Start It Up. https://medium.com/swlh/start-where-you-are-use-what-you-have-do-what-you-can-d41ddd58192d

Hereford, Z. (n.d.). "Tips for overcoming adversity." Essential Life Skills. https://www.essentiallifeskills.net/overcoming-adversity.html

Houston, E. (2020, December 28). "What is goal setting and how to do it well." Positive Psychology. https://positivepsychology.com/goal-setting/

"How can I speed up my metabolism?" (2020, October 26). NHS. https://www.nhs.uk/live-well/healthy-weight/metabolism-and-weight loss/

"How to transform your body (hard truths)." (2018, May 14). Team Body Project. https://teambodyproject.com/uncategorized/transform-body-hard-truths/

"It's not rocket science! The surprisingly simple formula for real weight loss." (n.d.). The Fitness Center. https://tfcoflilburn.com/its-not-rocket-science-the-surprisingly-simple-formula-for-real-weight loss/

Kelly, C. (n.d.). "Why you should always have a plan b in life & in business." Camden Kelly. https://camden-kelly.com/why-you-should-always-have-a-plan-b-in-life-in-business/

Kruse, K. (2016, March 7). "The 80/20 rule and how it can change your life." Forbes. https://www.forbes.com/sites/kevinkruse/2016/03/07/80-20-rule/?sh=twelve9467c03814

Lawler, M. (2021, May 18). "What is self-care and why is it so important for your health?" Everyday Health. https://www.everydayhealth.com/self-care/

Lenson, E. (2018, April 26). "Courage in adversity." Australian Academic Press. https://www.australianacademicpress.com.au/aap_blog/post/courage-in-adversity

Lim, S. (2018, September 5). "How to review your life: The 4 great methods to evaluate your life." Stunning Motivation. https://stunningmotivation.com/review-your-life/

"Losing weight is not rocket science." (n.d.). Ke Wynn Medical Fitness Center. http://www.kewynnpt.com/losing-weight-is-not-rocket-science/

Marcelo, G. (n.d.). "BJJ fanatics improve your skills." BJJ Heroes. https://www.bjjheroes.com/techniques/bow-and-arrow-standard-choke-from-back

Marcie. (n.d.). "How to keep your plans simple—and doable!" https://drmarcie.com/how-to-keep-your-plans-simple-and-doable/

Matt, T. (n.d.). "The cold truth about the diet industry in America." Life Hack. https://www.lifehack.org/520861/the-cold-truth-about-the-diet-industry-america

Mental Health Foundation. (n.d.). "How to manage and reduce stress." https://www.mentalhealth.org.uk/publications/how-manage-and-reduce-stress

Mind. (2017, October). "Mental health problems – an introduction." https://www.mind.org.uk/information-support/types-of-mental-health-problems/mental-health-problems-introduction/self-care/

Murray, L. (2017, April 26). "Keeping your courage in the face of adversity." Athena Leadership Academy. https://www.athenacoaching.com.au/keeping-your-courage-in-the-face-of-adversity/

National Eating Disorders Collaboration. (n.d.). "Disordered eating & dieting." https://nedc.com.au/eating-disorders/eating-disorders-explained/disordered-eating-and-dieting/

Nietzsche, Friedrich. (1990). Maxims and arrows. *Twilight of the Idols* (Penguin Classics ed.). (R. J. Hollingdale, Trans.). (Original work published 1889). Penguin.

"Overcoming adversity: The most overlooked leadership skill?" (2019, June 7). Core Process. https://www.coreprocess.co/overcoming-adversity-leadership-skill/

Palmer, M. (2013, May 21). "5 facts about body image." Amplify. http://amplifyyourvoice.org/u/marioapalmer/2013/05/21/byob-be-your-own-beautiful

Perkins, H. (2015, October twelve). "10 things no one tells you about transforming your body." Women's Health. https://www.womenshealthmag.com/fitness/a19917622/10-things-no-one-tells-you-about-transforming-your-body/

Pettit, M. (2020, May 4). "The power of writing down your goals, and how to do it." Thrive Global. https://thriveglobal.com/stories/the-power-of-writing-down-your-goals-and-how-to-do-it/

Pettit, M. (2020, March 4). "The importance of writing down your goals." Lucemi Consulting. https://lucemiconsulting.co.uk/writing-down-your-goals/

Radhakrishnan, R. (2020, February 9). "What are the 5 main food groups?" Medicine Net. https://www.medicinenet.com/what_are_the_5_main_food_groups/article.htm

Roomer, J. (2019, November twelve). "Why you need a strong commitment to your goals if you want to succeed." Personal Growth Lab. https://medium.com/personal-growth-lab/why-you-need-strong-commitment-to-a-goal-if-you-want-to-succeed-c5b095b5075f

Russo, A. (2015, September 16). "Best advice I ever got: Always have a plan." Inc. https://www.inc.com/young-entrepreneur-council/best-advice-i-ever-got-always-have-a-plan.html

Schenck, L. (n.d.). "Hardiness: Courage to thrive in the face of adversity." Mindfulness Muse. https://www.mindfulnessmuse.com/positive-psychology/hardiness-courage-to-thrive-in-the-face-of-adversity

Scott, M. (2021, June 11). "How overcoming adversity can shape you into a better person." Inspiyr. https://inspiyr.com/strength-courage-overcoming-adversity/

Severson, A. (2019, April 1). "Testosterone levels by age." Healthline. https://www.healthline.com/health/low-testosterone/testosterone-levels-by-age

Smith-Douglas, V. (n.d.). "8 things that hard workers do that sets them apart." Fairygodboss. https://fairygodboss.com/career-topics/what-does-hard-work-mean

Spritzler, F. (2020, March 9). "Do 'diets' really just make you fatter?" Healthline. https://www.healthline.com/nutrition/do-diets-make-you-gain-weight

Stevenson, T. (2019, October 24). "If you want to be successful, you need to work hard." Medium. https://medium.com/swlh/if-you-want-to-be-successful-you-need-to-work-hard-41af962b6ed0

Thornton, E. (2016, April 6). "The principles of objectivity can help you think smarter." Psychology Today. https://www.psychologytoday.com/za/blog/the-objective-leader/201604/the-principles-objectivity-can-help-you-think-smarter

"Transformation coach Adam Grayston to women around the world – Diets are making you bigger, not slimmer." (2021, January 11). EIN Presswire. https://www.einnews.com/pr_news/534327899/transformation-coach-adam-grayston-to-women-around-the-world-diets-are-making-you-bigger-not-slimmer

Tsenase, W. (2019, October 3). "3 keys to getting the results you want in life." Addicted to Success. https://

addicted2success.com/life/3-keys-to-getting-the-results-you-want-in-life/

"U.S. weight loss & diet control market report 2021." (2021, March 26). Business Wire. https://www.businesswire.com/news/home/20210326005126/en/U.S.-Weight-Loss-Diet-Control-Market-Report-2021-Market-Reached-a-Record-78-Billion-in-2019-but-Suffered-a-21-Decline-in-2020-Due-to-COVID-19---Forecast-to-2025---ResearchAndMarkets.com.

Wadhwa, H. (n.d.). "Change your mindset, transform your life." Hitendra Wadhwa. https://www.hitendra.com/hitendras-articles/change-your-mindset-transform-your-life

Waehner, P. (2020, May 26). "10 reasons why it's hard to lose weight." Very Well Fit. https://www.verywellfit.com/reasons-its-hard-to-lose-weight-twelve31540

Waehner, P. (2019, June 24). "Situations that sabotage your weight loss." Very Well Fit. https://www.verywellfit.com/weight loss-sabotage-p2-twelve31609

"Why people procrastinate: The psychology and causes of procrastination." (n.d.). Solving Procrastination. https://solvingprocrastination.com/why-people-procrastinate/

Williams, J. (n.d.). "Session 5 - future pacing." Academic Life Coaching. https://www.academiclifecoaching.com/coaching/parent-guide/future-pacing/

"Would you love to be part of the 5% that become super successful at losing weight and keeping it off?" (n.d.). Women Who Conquer. https://www.womenwhoconquer.co.uk/coaching44853550

Zoella (2020, January 10). "Twelve ways to make yourself a priority." https://zoella.co.uk/2020/01/10/twelve-ways-to-make-yourself-a-priority-2/

"10 weight loss myths." (2018, August 2). NHS. https://www.nhs.uk/live-well/healthy-weight/ten-weight loss-myths/

Printed in Poland
by Amazon Fulfillment
Poland Sp. z o.o., Wrocław